A Self-Instructional Guide:

PRINCIPLES OF BIOPSY

by

Thomas H. Morton, Jr., DDS, MSD
Robert J. Whitacre, MS, DDS
John D. Gehrig, DDS, MSD

A Self-Instructional Guide:

PRINCIPLES OF BIOPSY

Third Edition

(ISBN #0-89939-081-1)

AUTHORS

THOMAS H. MORTON, JR., DDS, MS, Department of Oral Medicine, Department of Oral Biology, Division of Oral Pathology, School of Dentistry, University of Washington, Seattle, Washington.

ROBERT J. WHITACRE, MS, DDS, Educational Consultant, Department of Oral and Maxillofacial Surgery, School of Dentistry, University of Washington, Seattle, Washington.

JOHN D. GEHRIG, DDS, MSD, Department of Oral and Maxillofacial Surgery, School of Dentistry, University of Washington, Seattle, Washington.

Illustrated by

Joan Hohl, D. Scott Phillips, DDS
and Dick Eidal, DDS

This book is one of a series of self-instructional textbooks designed to teach concepts of oral surgery and related disciplines to dental students, dental practitioners and dental auxiliaries. The series title of **A Self-Instructional Guide to Oral Surgery in General Dentistry** was formerly used to describe this series; however, many individuals outside of the specialty of oral surgery have expressed a desire to expand the titles of these books to facilitate transmission of this material in their areas. This series includes the following self-instructional book titles:

1. **Instruments Used for Oral Surgery**
2. **The Removal of Teeth**
3. **Medications Used in Oral Surgery**
4. **Surgical Complications**
5. **Dental Asepsis**
6. **Assessment of and Surgery for Impacted Third Molars**
7. **Pre-Prosthetic Surgery**
8. **Principles of Biopsy**
9. **Diagnosis and Treatment of Odontogenic Infections**

published by

Stoma Press, Inc.

13231 42nd Avenue NE
Seattle, WA 98125
(206) 365-2665

Typeset By
CASTEEL TYPESETTING
18316 1st NE
Seattle, WA 98155
(206) 363-9054

Printed By
ATOMIC PRESS
1421 N 34th
Seattle, WA
(206) 632-0550

EDITORS

JAMES R. HOOLEY, DDS, Dean and Professor of Oral and Maxillofacial Surgery, School of Dentistry, University of California at Los Angeles, Los Angeles, California.

ROBERT J. WHITACRE, MS, DDS, Educational Consultant, Department of Oral and Maxillofacial Surgery, School of Dentistry, University of Washington, Seattle, Washington.

EDITORIAL CONSULTANTS

TABLE OF CONTENTS

MESSAGE TO LEARNER

When reading a standard textbook, it is often difficult for you to know exactly what the important content is. It is difficult to separate areas that are essential for you to understand from those that are nice to know. You may often have thought you knew the material but could not apply it when presented with the clinical situation. You may also have had a problem during examinations when instructors asked you questions that were **not** covered in your reading.

In writing this book, considerable time and effort have been invested in creating a feedback system for you to monitor your learning progress. We have included a section termed "overview and objectives" which states the essential kinds of performances or knowledge you can expect to gain from reading the contents and completing the study exercises. We have included a **"Pre-Test"** for each unit. The "Pre-Test" is intended to show you what you don't know about the content of the unit. It is difficult for you to see learning take place unless you have both a "before" and "after" demonstration. You should retake the pre-tests following completion of each unit.

The **study exercises** are designed for different levels of learning. The **first level** of study exercises are of the "fill in the blank" type. The blanks usually include "key" words or phrases taken from the content preceding the study exercise.

The **second level** of study exercises is designed as problem-solving tasks. Generally these take a small piece of a larger concept and allow you to focus your attention on mastery of the piece. Learning one piece at a time is similar to learning your multiplication tables. The small pieces are then assimilated into larger concepts which you can learn with ease.

The **third level** of questions are simulations of clinical problems that you will be faced with in treating patients. Having completed the previous study exercises, you should be able to adequately cope with these. These are the most important study exercises because they resemble the real world of dentistry. Through adequate analysis and planning, complications or surprises during surgery can be greatly reduced. These are similar to "story problems" in mathematics.

The study exercises are **extremely important** and you should take the time to **write the answers** in the blanks or spaces provided. You may be tempted to mentally answer the questions or skip them entirely to save time. You will **retain more of the information** you have read with much **less effort** if you take the time to write out the answers as you proceed. Considerable research in self-instructional design and learning has shown the importance of answering such study questions.

Even though the content in this book appears large, by no means did we intend to present the entire field of oral pathology and surgical biopsy procedures. We intend this book to be your "starter kit," and strongly encourage you to obtain other reference books, journals, and materials to supplement topics not discussed in detail.

Although we have had considerable input from many people in writing this book, we by no means imply that techniques, instruments or concepts are the "only way." Your oral surgeon or instructors may wish to deviate from the methods described, especially with regard to specific clinical situations.

RECOMMENDED ENTRY KNOWLEDGE

This book assumes you have had previous training in the areas listed below and it may be beneficial for you to review this material as we discuss the various topics in relation to management of oral lesions.

1. Basic knowledge of normal oral anatomy including proper diagnostic techniques for a complete oral examination and the skills required to detect an oral lesion.
2. Course in Oral Pathology and access to a current oral pathology textbook.
3. Training in how to obtain a thorough review of your patient's health history.
4. Working clinical knowledge of osseous and soft tissue anatomy and morphology of the head, neck and oral cavity.
5. Basic oral surgery techniques including:
   a. Incision techniques.
   b. Suture techniques.
   c. Post-operative management skills.
   d. Post-operative medications.

OVERVIEW AND OBJECTIVES

The purpose of this book is to assist you in developing an operational system for performing or referring surgical biopsies; preparing data and specimens for your pathologist; interpreting the results of the pathologist's report; and selecting the appropriate treatment option. Unit I discusses how to determine whether a surgical specimen is necessary. Unit II describes the various types of surgical techniques and how they should be modified for particular lesions and locations. Unit III presents a system for evaluating the "degree of difficulty" in obtaining a surgical specimen and using this evaluation as criteria for referral. Unit IV develops a system for patient management after interpretation of your pathologist's report.

UNIT I—GENERAL MANAGEMENT PHILOSOPHY FOR ORAL LESIONS

As the title implies, this unit is designed to provide you with a workable general management philosophy for managing the lesions you will encounter during your treatment of patients. Although the actual number of oral cancers appears low (5 percent of all body cancers), an early diagnosis by first-line health care personnel leads to a great increase in the favorable prognosis for your patients.

After completing this unit, you will:

1. Define the term "biopsy."

2. Determine the need for biopsy from clinical descriptions and photographs of oral conditions, and then state specific rules why a surgical procedure is or is not indicated.

3. Describe your non-surgical treatment options for treating oral lesions.

4. Describe the necessary course of action when you have detected a lesion for which you have a high suspicion of malignancy.

5. When given any oral lesion and a brief history, choose the correct avenue for managing the patient's lesion and decide when surgical removal of a tissue specimen is necessary.

UNIT II—SURGICAL REMOVAL OF A TISSUE SPECIMEN

This unit discusses steps you should take before surgery; general surgical principles for incisional, excisional and bone biopsies; site selection and surgical modifications required for particular lesions. It also discusses care of the specimen during and after surgery and how to complete the request for histopathologic examination.

After completing this unit, you will:

1. Describe the necessary data you should record **before** surgery.

2. Describe how you should discuss this procedure with your patient before surgery to avoid needless anguish.

3. Describe the **general rules** that serve as guidelines for planning and performing the surgical removal of a tissue specimen:
    a. Size
    b. Appearance
    c. Adequate section
    d. Location
    e. Anesthesia
    f. Anatomical considerations

4. Describe the following surgical methods for removing a tissue specimen and state the indications and contraindications for each.
    a. Excisional biopsy
    b. Incisional biopsy
    c. Bone biopsy
    d. Aspiration biopsy
    e. Punch biopsy
    f. Exfoliative cytology
    g. Curettage biopsy

5. Describe the general technique for removing a soft tissue specimen (including specific instruments used).

6. Describe the general technique for removing a radiolucent lesion from bone (including specific instruments used).

7. State the four basic rules for site selection as related to surgical outline and position relative to underlying anatomy.

8. Given intraoral photographs of oral lesions, correctly draw the outline for your biopsy according to the four general guidelines identified in objective II-4.
9. Describe and diagram the basic outline for a "normal" excisional biopsy. Include dimensions for the borders of normal tissue required.
10. Describe two modifications of the usual excisional biopsy outline and indications for their use.
11. Given intraoral photographs or diagrams of oral lesions requiring excisional biopsy, determine whether your outline should be normal or modified. If modified, state the modification needed and why this is necessary.
12. Describe and diagram the usual shape for incisional biopsies. Your description should include a description of the type of sample, plus the amount of normal margin usually required, and size of lesion for which this is used.
13. Describe the usual modifications for the basic incisional technique. Give an example where each should be used.
14. Describe how the physical properties of a lesion, including, (1) definition of margins; (2) surface characteristics; (3) depth of extension; (4) quality of tissue; (5) pigmentation; (6) vascularity; (7) soft tissue or bone; and (8) growth rate, influence the use and the design of the incisional technique.
15. Given intraoral photographs of lesions, analyze all physical properties and state whether modifications of the basic technique are necessary. If so, describe the necessary modification and why this should be done.
16. Given intraoral photographs and a brief clinical history, state the malignant potential for the lesions shown.
17. Describe how you should handle the biopsy specimen after surgery.
18. Properly complete a request for microscopic examination of tissue by your oral pathologist.

UNIT III—EVALUATION OF DEGREE OF DIFFICULTY AS A CRITERION FOR REFERRAL

This unit is designed to build your discriminating skills so you can learn to evaluate those factors that modify the difficulty of obtaining a surgical specimen. Once these factors are evaluated, you arc in a better position to determine the degree of difficulty, and use this information as a basis for referring your patients to a specialist.

Following completion of this unit, you will:

1. Analyze simulated clinical cases using the summary sheet for evaluation criteria and the lesion evaluation and record sheet, and then rate each factor for degree of difficulty.

2. State the reasons for referral or treatment of a lesion, based on your analysis of the case.

UNIT IV—WHAT TO DO WITH YOUR PATHOLOGIST'S REPORT

This unit is designed to help you in decisions concerning the course of treatment required after microscopic examination of the tissue specimen. Selection of the proper referral source is essential for prompt management of malignant lesions. Delay decreases the prognosis for your patient.

Following completion of this unit, you will:

1. Describe and explain the course of action if your clinical impression of a lesion is that it is more malignant than described in the pathologist's report.

2. Given examples of pathologist's reports, identify for each whether the lesion is neoplastic or non-neoplastic and the specific subdivisions of these categories. (You may use the "terminology" section of the book for this.)

3. Select the correct treatment modality(ies) for any lesion based on the pathologist's report.

4. State what you should keep in mind when informing your patient about a diagnosis of cancer.

GENERAL OBJECTIVE FOR THIS BOOK

Given clinical photographs, clinical descriptions of non-visual data, and health history information, you will analyze any lesion, decide on the appropriate action required, and state why. You will be asked to follow the treatment through the receipt of the pathology report and describe your actions from there. All data and decisions should be placed on the evaluation and treatment record. You should include a description of the type of biopsy sample required, how you would approach the surgery, what to do with the specimen, completion of the pathology request form, interpretation of the pathology report, and your final decision for action. Your criteria for decisions should be based on the stated criteria in this book.

UNIT I

GENERAL MANAGEMENT PHILOSOPHY FOR ORAL LESIONS

Pre-Test
Introduction
General Treatment Philosophy
Detection of an Oral Lesion
Criteria for Biopsy
Guidelines for Surgical Removal of Tissue
Treatment Options for Oral Lesions

PRE-TEST—Unit I

- *Cover answers on Page 13.*
- *Answer the following questions.*
- *Compare your answers with those provided. If responses are correct, proceed to Unit II. If only some were correct, you will benefit from studying this unit. Proceed to Page 14.*

Questions:

1. *Considering a general practice of 1,500 to 2,000 patients, you, as the dentist in charge, might expect to be involved in the detection, diagnoses, referral, or treatment of how many cancerous lesions of the head and neck (general order of magnitude based on average statistics)?*

   a. 1 every 10 years
   b. 1 every year
   c. 10 every year
   d. 100 every year

	True	*False*	
2.	________	________	*A biopsy procedure is usually performed to establish a definitive diagnosis of cancer.*

3. *For each of the lesions described below, state whether your first action after detection should be to surgically remove a tissue specimen for microscopic examination (check the appropriate column and give your reason).*

Biopsy Needed Now by You or a Specialist	*Do Not Biopsy At This Time*	
☐	☐	a. See Color Plate III, Fig. 59. The lesions on the lateral border of the tongue have developed over many years as a result of irritation during chewing. Why?________________________________

Biopsy Needed Now by You or a Specialist	Do Not Biopsy At This Time	
☐	☐	b. Your tentative diagnosis of the elevated structures on the buccal mucosa approximating the linea alba is that these are Fordyce's Granules. Why?__________
☐	☐	c. You have detected what appears to be bilateral red lesions on the lateral border of the tongue in the posterior area distal to the mandibular second molar region. Why?__________
☐	☐	d. You have detected a 5 mm. irritation fibroma (fibroma durum) on the buccal mucosa. This lesion has a long history of being irritated during mastication. Why?__________
☐	☐	e. You have detected a lesion for which you can find no apparent etiology. Why?__________
☐	☐	f. You have detected a lesion which has shown a slow enlargement under your patient's denture and has not responded to conservative treatment. Why?__________

4. For the following clinical cases, give the number that would specify the correct way this situation should be managed at this stage.
   1 = observe lesion for 7-14 days
   2 = non-surgical treatment for 7-14 days
   3 = laboratory tests
   4 = high suspicion of cancer (refer to specialist immediately)
   5 = decision to remove tissue for diagnosis now

   a. ______ See Plate II, Fig. 47. Mr. A.J., a 42-year-old salesman, after eating a particularly tough steak three days ago, noticed an ulcer 4 mm in diameter on the lateral border of his tongue. It has been painful and is sore whenever he eats, talks, or otherwise moves his tongue. How would you manage this case? Explain.
   ____
   ____

   b. ______ See Plate I, Fig. 26. Mr. O.P., a 26-year-old black student, two days ago noticed a red, swollen, painful lump, approximately 1 cm in diameter on his left anterior palate opposite a cariously exposed maxillary right first premolar. He develops a bad taste in his mouth when he presses on it with his tongue. How would you manage this patient's problem? Explain. __________
   ____

   c. ______ See Plate II, Fig. 50. Mrs. H.G., a 32-year-old housewife, presents to your office with a 9 mm lump in her right lower lip of about two years' duration. It is usually painless, but when bitten, enlarges and gets slightly tender. Occasionally it bursts, drains, and recedes to almost nothing. How would you manage this patient's problem? Explain.__________
   ____

PRE-TEST—Unit 1, Answers

1. *b—one every year*

2. *False*

3. a. *Biopsy needed—lesion is interfering with local function.*

   b. *Do not biopsy—normal anatomical variants are not biopsied unless they interfere with local function.*

   c. *Do not biopsy—you are probably seeing inflamed folliate papillae. These are normal anatomical structures.*

   d. *Biopsy needed—lesion is interfering with local function.*

   e. *Biopsy needed—histopathologic examination can be of assistance in arriving at a diagnosis and determining treatment.*

   f. *Biopsy needed—lesion does not respond to conservative non-surgical treatment.*

4. a. __1__ *Your tentative diagnosis is traumatic ulcer. Wait 7-14 days; it may resolve.*

   b. __2__ *The lesion is probably related to a periapical abscess of the cariously involved tooth. The lesion will most likely resolve following root canal therapy.*

   c. __5__ *This lesion is interfering with local function and should be removed.*

CONTENT FOR UNIT I

GENERAL MANAGEMENT PHILOSOPHY FOR ORAL LESIONS

INTRODUCTION

In this book, we will develop the concept that "biopsy" is not merely a surgical technique for oral lesions. Rather, it entails a total patient management philosophy for oral lesions involving:

- adequate **data collection**
- competent **diagnostic skills**
- proper **surgical management**
- **evaluation and interpretation** of the pathologist's report
- comprehensive patient **follow-up**

The number of oral or head and neck lesions you might see among 2,000 patients a year may be considerable, since 80 percent of all skin cancers occur in the head and neck region. You will diagnose tori, geographic tongues, denture injury hyperplasia, decubitus ulcers, aphthous stomatitis, herpetic ulcerations, chemical burns, linea albas, abscesses, cysts, and many keratotic lesions. The keratotic lesions will require identification of the etiology, and the surgical removal of tissue may be required.

Of significant importance is the detection of head and neck cancer. Head and neck cancer frequently occurs in older, but otherwise healthy, individuals. Because of their good health, many of these patients do not see their physicians regularly. Therefore, physicians are often not in a good position to provide early diagnosis of oral and head and neck lesions. On the other hand, a thorough dental examination once or twice a year is a fairly common practice among this patient group.

Note: It is our responsibility as dentists to perform a careful head and neck examination of each patient and to coordinate proper management of any lesions that are detected during this process.

GENERAL TREATMENT PHILOSOPHY

The following discussion is meant to give you an overview of the general treatment philosophy for the treatment of any oral lesion.

Definition of Biopsy:

Biopsy is the removal of a representative section of living tissue from a lesion for microscopic examination and diagnosis.

Purpose of Biopsy:

- To determine whether a lesion is an inflammatory, reactive, systemic, or neoplastic process.
- To determine whether a neoplastic process is malignant.
- If malignant, to type, grade, or stage the lesion to determine a prognosis.
- To formulate a specific treatment.

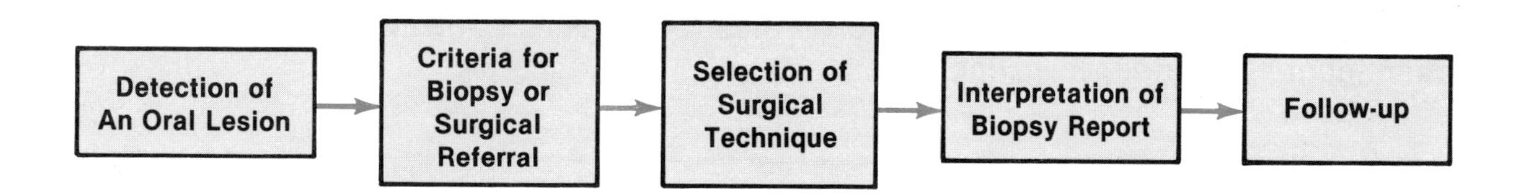

Figure I-1. Overview of a General Biopsy Procedure for Management of Lesions

DETECTION OF AN ORAL LESION

Need for Thorough Medical and Dental History

A thorough medical and dental history should be recorded for all patients. A thorough head and neck examination is also essential.

> **Example**
>
> The presence of a lesion in a patient with a previous history of malignancy may influence your decision to biopsy. Also, systemic disease processes, such as hyperparathyroidism, malnutrition, aging, etc., may give insight into possible oral changes and the need for biopsy.

Specific Data Collection

To recognize that a lesion is present, you need to distinguish between normal oral structures and pathological deviations from the normal, whether they be neoplastic, reactive, inflammatory, or developmental.

The following outline for detection and description of a lesion is essential for optimum communication with your pathologist and in the total management of the lesion, including treatment and prognosis.

✓ **You need to recognize normal:**

- Anatomy
- Color and Texture
- Function
- Radiographic appearance

✓ **You need to completely evaluate and record deviations from the normal by:**

- Palpation
- Oscultation
- Visual description
- Photographs
- Radiographic characteristics

✓ **All data must be adequately described in your patient's treatment record.**

The above diagnostic techniques are assumed knowledge for you at this time and will not be further elaborated on in this book. See list of references for more detail on these techniques.

STUDY EXERCISES—Treatment Philosophy

The biopsy procedure is more than a surgical technique. It involves a comprehensive management strategy involving:

1. Adequate ______________________ collection.
2. Competent ______________________ skills.
3. Proper ______________________ management.
4. Evaluation and interpretation of the ______________________'s report.
5. Comprehensive patient ______________________.

You as a dentist, are in a better position to diagnose head and neck cancer in older healthy patients because ______________________
____
______________________.

Biopsy is the ______________________
______________________.

The purpose of a biopsy is to:

a. Determine whether a lesion is______________________, ______________________, ______________________ or ______________________.

b. Determine if the neoplastic process is ______________________.

c. If a lesion is malignant, to: ______________, ______________, or ______________ the lesion to determine a ______________________.

d. To formulate a specific ______________________.

Figure I-1 describes the overall management for oral lesions detected in your office. What are the five important steps? (Each will be developed further in subsequent text and study exercises).

a. ______________________
b. ______________________
c. ______________________
d. ______________________
e. ______________________

CRITERIA FOR BIOPSY

The key decision you must make when you first detect a lesion is to decide **whether** to remove tissue for microscopic examination. You should check the following situations or conditions and rule out those conditions which do not usually require surgical removal of tissue.

✓ **DO NOT biopsy normal anatomic structures and developmental variants.**

- Inflamed lingual tonsils
- Leukoedema
- Fordyce granules
- Retrocuspid papillae
- Median rhomboid glossitis
- Linea alba
- Physiologic pigmentation
- Geographic tongue

✓ **DO NOT biopsy traumatic lesions which may first respond to removal of etiologic factors, especially tissue trauma caused by impingement of sharp tooth structures.**

✓ **DO NOT biopsy inflammatory lesions which may first respond to local treatments.**

- Periodontal abscess
- Periocoronitis
- Gingivitis

✓ **DO NOT biopsy a lesion that requires biopsy techniques beyond your realm of surgical ability.**

When Should You Remove Tissue for Microscopic Examination?

You should consider surgical removal of tissue for microscopic examination for any condition found in the oral cavity that is:

- A deviation from the normal anatomical structures; or
- Any inflammatory conditions which fail to respond to conservative treatment,
- All lesions which have no obvious or apparent etiological basis or pose a problem in diagnosis or treatment

GUIDELINES FOR SURGICAL REMOVAL OF TISSUE (BIOPSY)

DO biopsy lesions that do not respond to local treatment within 7-14 days:

- After removal of local irritant,
- Non-healing of an apparent inflammatory or infectious process when treated with antibiotics or anti-inflammatory drugs.

DO biopsy lesions that interfere with local function:

- Irritation fibroma (fibroma durum) on buccal mucosa at occlusal line.
- Torus mandibularus undergoing chronic trauma.
- Hyperplastic tuberosity

DO biopsy lesions that show slow enlargement or sudden growth (bone or soft tissue).

DO biopsy lesions that have no apparent etiology.

DO biopsy lesions that are long-standing, white or red (such as in chronic tobacco use).

DO biopsy lesions that are pigmented or angiomatous.

DO biopsy radiolucent (osteolytic) or radiopaque (osteoblastic) lesions in bone which are not periapical.

DO biopsy lesions that are associated with pain, parasthesia, or anesthesia of unknown etiology.

DO biopsy lesions that are deep masses within the muscle of the tongue, buccal mucosa or lip.

STUDY EXERCISES—Indications and Contraindications for Biopsy

For each of the clinical cases described below, state whether you **should** *or* **should not** *remove tissue for microscopic examination. State also the guideline upon which your decision was based. Plate and Figure references are to the color photographs provided at the end of this chapter.*

Should	Should Not	
☐	☐	1. *See Plate II, Fig. 55. This white palatal lesion has remained after the patient quit smoking one month ago. It has not responded to other conservative treatment.* *Guideline:* ________________
☐	☐	2. *See Plate I, Fig. 28. You have just constructed a temporary crown for the mandibular right second molar. The lesion on the lateral border of the tongue has been present for about three days.* *Guideline:* ________________
☐	☐	3. *See Plate II, Fig. 49. The patient has been aware of this lesion for about one month and claims it "moves around" on his tongue.* *Guideline:* ________________
☐	☐	4. *See Plate III, Fig. 73. A former professional athlete who chews tobacco presents with this lesion.* *Guideline:* ________________
☐	☐	5. *See Plate I, Fig. 2. Your patient has been aware of this lesion for many years. The lesion is occasionally traumatized during mastication.* *Guideline:* ________________
☐	☐	6. *See Plate I, Fig. 27. Your patient complains of pain in the mandibular left canine. He said he had to place an aspirin next to the tooth in order to get to sleep last night.* *Guideline:* ________________
☐	☐	7. *See Plate I, Fig. 20. Your patient claims this palatal mass with a large central ulcer developed over the last two weeks. Your patient also complains of nasal stuffiness.* *Guideline:* ________________
☐	☐	8. *See Plate III, Fig. 64. This lesion has persisted for two weeks following periodontal therapy.* *Guideline:* ________________
☐	☐	9. *See Plate III, Fig. 74. Your patient was not aware of this lesion until you pointed it out to her. She has warts on her fingers which she habitually chews.* *Guideline:* ________________
☐	☐	10. *See Plate III, Fig. 67. This lesion has been present ever since the patient was a child. He also has a "port wine" nevus on the left cheek.* *Guideline* ________________

STUDY EXERCISES—Answers to Clinical Cases

	Should	Should Not	Guideline:
1.	☒	☐	*White lesion does not respond to local conservative treatment.*
2.	☐	☒	*Traumatic ulcer should respond to your local therapy.*
3.	☐	☒	*Do not biopsy geographic tongue.*
4.	☐	☒	*Snuff keratosis may first respond to local therapy.*
5.	☒	☐	*This lesion is interfering with local function.*
6.	☐	☒	*This aspirin burn will probably resolve within 14 days.*
7.	☒	☐	*Lesion shows sudden growth.*
8.	☒	☐	*Lesion does not respond to conservative therapy.*
9.	☒	☐	*Verruca vulgaris lesions are the result of a viral infection which may continue to spread to other areas. This lesion will not respond to local treatment and may interfere with local function.*
10.	☐	☒	*This hemangioma is a developmental variant (also, surgery for conditions of this nature is usually beyond the ability of most general practitioners).*

TREATMENT OPTIONS FOR ORAL LESIONS

The following diagram may be useful in clarifying your treatment options once you have detected an oral lesion.

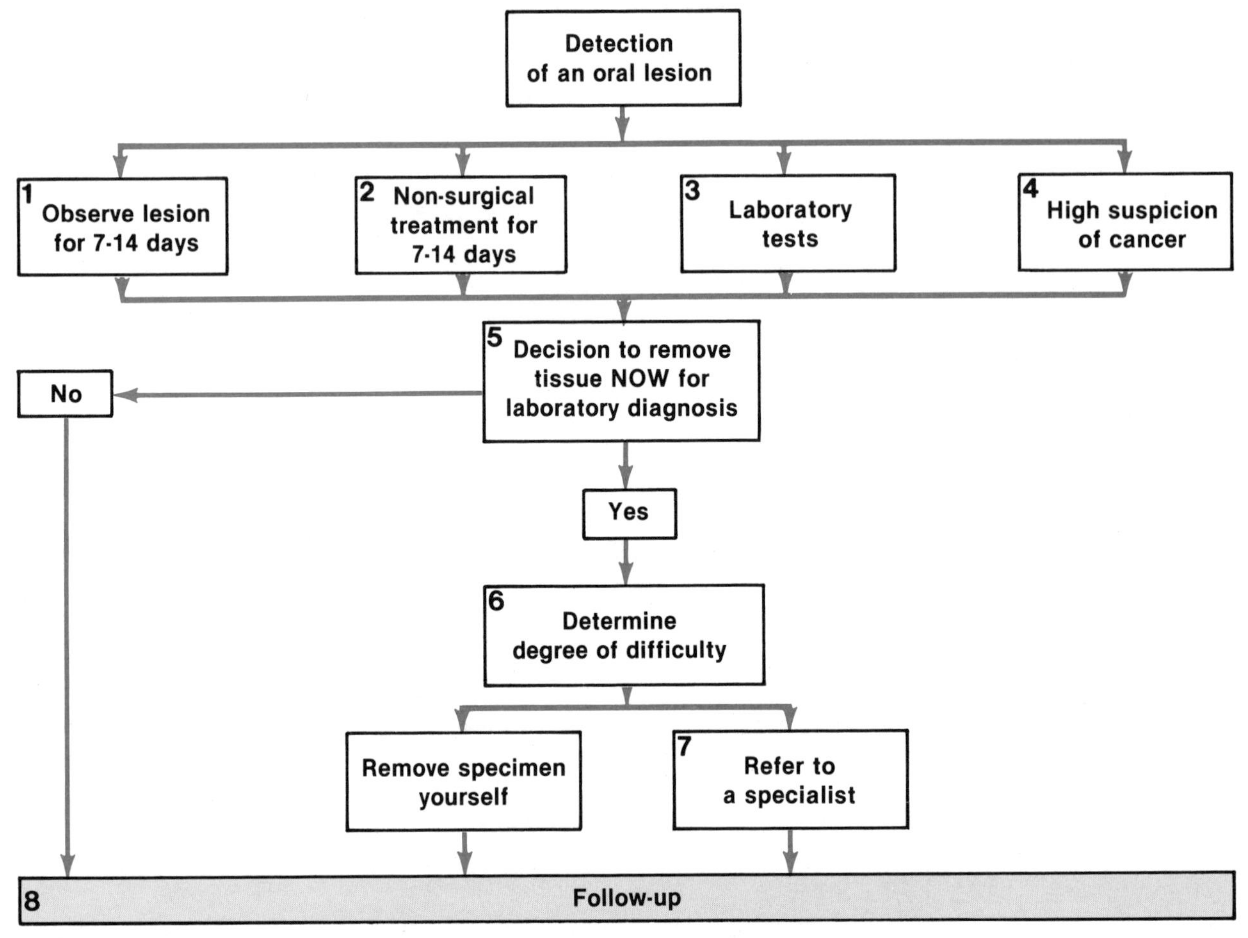

Figure I-2. Treatment Options for Oral Lesions

Figure I-2 shows a flow chart of your treatment options after the detection of an oral lesion. It divides your options into first, non-surgical modalities, then into methods requiring the removal of tissue for microscopic examination. It then emphasizes that whether you use non-surgical or surgical treatment, adequate follow-up is essential. The following descriptions provide specific examples for each of your treatment options.

1. **Observe for 7-14 days:**
   - Areas of trauma, chemical or local irritation after etiologic factor(s) are removed.
   - Red, or ulcerated areas in smokers.
   - To ensure the healing process is on-going.
   - To compare any possible changes at a future date.

2. **Non-surgical treatment for lesions that may respond to:**
   - Antibiotic therapy.
   - Lavage.
   - Repair of sharp, failing restorations.
   - Lining of prosthetic devices.
   - Removal of external factors such as cigarette smoking or tobacco chewing.

3. **You may wish to perform lab tests before and/or with the surgical removal of tissue to help determine a working diagnosis. Useful tests include:**

    - Blood tests
    - Culture and sensitivity
    - Glucose tolerance tests for diabetes mellitus
    - Skin tests for allergy
    - Radiographic surveys
    - Dietary tests

4. **Lesions for which you have a high suspicion of malignancy when you first observe them require that you submit tissue to the pathologist immediately, or refer the patient immediately to a specialist. Waiting 7-14 days may reduce the prognosis for your patient.**

5. **If a lesion responds to local therapy, the decision is not to biopsy.** This, however, does not preclude a follow-up at regular intervals.

    The decision should be to remove tissue for microscopic examination if:

    - a lesion does not repond to local treatment
    - shows changes in shape, size, and coloration
    - is considered malignant

6. **At this time you must decide if the surgical technique required to facilitate the proper diagnosis of the lesion is within your ability.** If so, you proceed with the biopsy procedure which will include:

    - the removal of the tissue
    - the completion of request for laboratory study
    - the submission of the tissue to a pathologist
    - the complete reading and understanding of the diagnostic report
    - complete follow-up

7. **If the required surgical technique is beyond your ability, or if a more extensive surgical procedure is required after your initial biopsy, you should refer your patient to an oral and maxillofacial surgeon.**

8. **Whether or not you remove the tissue specimen yourself, you should be informed on the disposition of your patient and should maintain your patient on long-term follow-up.**

STUDY EXERCISES—*Treatment Options*

For each of the following clinical cases and using the management system previously discussed, describe how each case should be managed and the specific reasons for your decision.

Case:

1. *See Plate II, Fig. 47. A 42-year-old white salesman noticed a lesion on the posterior lateral border of his tongue. Upon questioning, you discover he had had a difficult time chewing a tough steak about three days ago. His tongue has been sore since that time.*
   Treatment Decision: ______________________________
   Reasons for Decision: ______________________________
   ____
   ____
   ____

2. *See Plate II, Fig. 48. A 26-year-old black student noticed a red, swollen, painful swelling on the anterior left side of the palate, opposite a cariously involved maxillary right first premolar. He develops a bad taste in his mouth when he presses on the lesion with his tongue.*
   Treatment Decision: ______________________________
   Reasons for Decision: ______________________________
   ____
   ____

3. *See Plate II, Fig. 49. You have noticed a slightly different appearance of the tongue of your new patient, a 38-year-old banking executive. The lesion apears as a white line around an erythematous patch. She has no symptoms associated with the lesion, although she says the lesion moves around on her tongue and has been there for as long as she can recall.*
   Treatment Decision: ______________________________
   Reasons for Decision: ______________________________
   ____
   ____

4. *See Plate II, Fig. 50. A 32-year-old housewife presents to your office with a 9 mm lump in her left lower lip. She says she has had this problem for over two years and that it occasionally gets larger, bursts, drains, and recedes to almost nothing.*
   Treatment Decision: ______________________________
   Reasons for Decision: ______________________________
   ____
   ____

5. *See Plate II, Fig. 51. A 56-year-old computer business executive, presents to you with this lesion. He is an active smoker (two packs/day) and wears complete dentures. He noticed the "white patches" under his denture last week and thought he should call you. The lesions measure 3 x 3 mm and 8 x 11 mm.*
   Treatment Decision: ______________________________
   Reasons for Decision: ______________________________
   ____
   ____

STUDY QUESTIONS—Answers

Case #1—assuming the patient snagged his tongue on the sharp molar while eating the steak, you would probably smooth off the sharp edges of the molar and observe the results for 7-14 days. At that time, you should re-evaluate the condition. Treatment = observe for 7-14 days.

Case #2—vitality tests indicate tooth #12 is non-vital. You would probably do root canal therapy on #12; then observe the course of the lesion. Treatment = non-surgical treatment.

Case #3—this lesion presents the signs of geographic tongue. You would decide biopsy is not appropriate. This condition is a normal anatomical variation. Treatment = do not surgically remove.

Case #4—this lesion should be removed for biopsy.

Case #5—first you should adjust the denture, wait for 7-14 days, then if the lesion does not resolve, remove a specimen for histopathological evaluation.

UNIT II

SURGICAL REMOVAL OF A TISSUE SPECIMEN

Pre-Test
Preparation for Surgery
General Surgical Principles for Biopsy
Site Selection and Surgical Modifications
Care and Handling of the Specimen Following Surgery
Completion of the Request for Laboratory Study Form

PRE-TEST—Unit II

- *Answer the following questions*
- *Compare your answers with those on page 27.*
- *If all your responses were correct, you have finished this unit.*
- *If only some of your responses were correct, you can profit from studying this unit.*

Questions:

1. *Describe the general rules that serve as guidelines for planning and performing the surgical removal of a tissue specimen that relate to:*
   a. *Size:* ____________________

   b. *Appearance:* ____________________

   c. *Adequate section:* ____________________

   d. *Location:* ____________________

   e. *Anesthesia:* ____________________

   f. *Anatomical considerations:* ____________________

2. *When would you use the following techniques?*
   a. *Excisional:* ____________________

   b. *Incisional:* ____________________

   c. *Aspiration or needle biopsy:* ____________________

3. *What essential precaution should be taken before incising into a radiolucent lesion in the jaw?* ____________________

4. *In the following illustration state whether it correctly or incorrectly depicts a proper outline for site selection. If the illustration shows an incorrect site selection or outline, state why it is incorrect.*

   a. *Correct ______ Incorrect ______*
   What's wrong? ______________________________

   b. *Correct ______ Incorrect ______*
   What's wrong? ______________________________

5. *In performing an excisional biopsy, you should normally think of a wedge-shaped eliptical incision that extends at least ______mm on either side of the lesion in the short axis and ______mm beyond the lesion in the long axis.*

6. *Often you will need to modify your usual outline for excisional biopsies. State: 1. what kinds of modifications you would most commonly encounter; 2. when you would modify; and 3. why?*

	Modification	*When Used?*	*Why?*
a.			
b.			

7. *Describe when you should biopsy a dark pigmented lesion or a vascular lesion by incisional technique. ______________________________*
   Why? ______________________________

8. *From looking at a lesion, what cues would tell you "you are dealing with a malignancy"?*
   a. ______________________________
   b. ______________________________
   c. ______________________________
   d. ______________________________

9. *From palpation of the lesion, what information would suggest "malignancy?"*
   a. ______________________________
   b. ______________________________

10. *Describe the accepted procedure for handling a tissue specimen after surgery:*
   ____

11. *How should you handle biopsy specimens if you have removed multiple specimens from the same lesion?______________________________*

12. *Examine the request for laboratory study below.*
    a. *Is this form adequately completed? Yes ____ No ____*
    b. *If not, check those line items that are unacceptable.*
    c. *Describe what is wrong with each numbered item:*

1.	______________	*8.*	______________
2.	______________	*9.*	______________
3.	______________	*10.*	______________
4.	______________	*11.*	______________
5.	______________	*12.*	______________
6.	______________	*13.*	______________
7.	______________		

REQUEST FOR LABORATORY STUDY

Unacceptable

1. ☐ **1. Patient's Name** John Mason **Age** **Sex** M **Race**

2. ☐ **2. Patient's Address**

3. ☐ **3. Doctor's Name** Wilson **Phone**

4. ☐ **4. Doctor's Address**

Number and Street

City **State** **Zip Code**

5. ☐ **5. Description of Lesion** (Include location, duration, size and color)

6. ☐ Lesion from oral cavity

6. Sketch of Lesion Site

7. ☐ **7. Associated Findings and Past History (including previous Biopsy Accession No.)**

Lesion was under denture

8. ☐ **8. Symptoms** Asymptomatic

9. ☐ **9. Radiographic Findings** ☐ **Radiographs Enclosed**

10. ☐ **10. Clinical Impression** Hyperkeratosis due to denture irretation

11. ☐ **11. Type of Biopsy:** ☐ **Incisional** ☐ **Excisional** ☐ **Aspiration** ☐ **Curettage** ☐ **Other**

12. ☐ **12. Date tissue removed:** 5/30/80 **Time:** ☐ **A.M.** ☐ **P.M.**

13. ☐ [signature]

13. Doctor's Signature

REV. 1/80

PRE-TEST—UNIT II, Answers

1. a. **Size:** *Excisional biopsy if lesion is less than 1.0 cm and usually an incisional biopsy if larger.*
   b. **Appearance:** *Choose the most suspicious area or areas for sampling.*
   c. **Adequate Section:** *Usually a thin deep section, including a normal border, is best.*
   d. **Location:** *Always annotate the specimen with a suture or straight pin before placing it in the formalin.*
   e. **Anesthesia:** *Use block anesthesia rather than local infiltration.*
   f. **Anatomical Considerations:** *Keep incisions within the long axis of major nerves and blood vessels.*
2. a. *If the lesion were less than 1.0 cm in size.*
   b. *If the lesion were greater than 1.0 cm in size.*
   c. *If the lesion was a radiolucent lesion in bone.*
3. *You should aspirate the lesion.*
4. a. *Incorrect. Incisions are perpendicular to the long axis of major nerves and blood vessels.*
   b. *Correct.*
5. *2 mm and 5 mm in this order*
6.

	Modification:	When used:	Why:
a.	*Increase lateral margins to 5 mm.*	*Pigmented or vascular lesions.*	*Must obtain adequate normal margins.*
b.	*Remove a block rather than a normal wedge.*	*Well circumscribed benign lesions.*	*To adequately remove all of the lesion.*

7. *NEVER*
   May cause severe (life threatening) bleeding problems or may "seed" pigmented lesion to other locations in the body.
8. a. *Fissuring or cracking*
   b. *Bleeds easily*
   c. *Areas of rapid growth*
   d. *Recurrence or persistence*
9. a. *Fixation to underlying tissue*
   b. *Induration*
10. *Properly annotated specimen should be blotted to remove excess blood and placed immediately into 10% formalin.*
11. *Identify each specimen distinctly, both on tissue and in request for laboratory study form. You may desire to place specimens in separate bottles.*
12. *This form is not adequately filled out.*
    1. *Need age and race.*
    2. *Need patient's address.*
    3. *Need doctor's full name and phone number.*
    4. *Need doctor's address.*
    5. *Inadequate description of drawing.*
    6. *Should have sketch of lesion.*
    7. *Usually more information is known about associated findings and patient's health history.*
    8. *Acceptable.*
    9. *State negative if negative.*
    10. *Acceptable.*
    11. *Must state the type of biopsy.*
    12. *Should check time*
    13. *Acceptable.*

CONTENT FOR UNIT II

SURGICAL REMOVAL OF A TISSUE SPECIMEN

PREPARATION FOR SURGERY

You have now proceeded in the biopsy technique to the point where removal of a tissue specimen is appropriate before definitive treatment can be initiated. Adequate data should be collected and recorded before surgery. This data is essential and can influence the diagnosis and extent of treatment. Proper surgical techniques insure the removal of an optimum tissue specimen. These techniques all involve basic principles, but often you must make slight modifications, depending upon the lesion involved.

After data collection, you must explain to your patient the need to surgically remove a tissue sample. You should be able to explain the need for this service in a manner that does not generate "cancer phobia."

Data Collection Prior To Surgery

- A thorough description of the lesion, including location, duration, size, shape, coloration and any radiographic findings.
- A summary of signs and symptoms.
- **A very accurate lymphadenopathy examination** (head and neck examination).
- Any associated findings and past history (this may include apparently insignificant past medical history).
- A clinical impression (differential diagnosis).

What To Tell Your Patients Prior To Biopsy

Needless worry and anguish may be caused by inappropriate use of words when you inform the patient of the need for a biopsy. Terms such as "tumor" or "growth" have a bad connotation to the lay person and may be interpreted as meaning cancer. The patient should be informed that he or she has a lesion which has not responded to therapy and, therefore, a tissue biopsy is indicated. Emphasis should be placed on the fact that a biopsy is just another diagnostic technique to better establish and facilitate treatment.

What steps must you take before removing a tissue specimen? ______________________

Information collected and recorded can be important in determining a definitive ________ ______________________ *and the extent of* ______________________ *necessary.*

The five main categories of data you should collect include:

a. ______________________

b. ______________________

c. ______________________

d. ______________________

e. ______________________

What should you tell your patient, and how should you phrase it, before removing a tissue specimen? ______________________

____

____

____

GENERAL SURGICAL PRINCIPLES FOR BIOPSY

The following general surgical principles should always be kept in mind when removing any lesion or portion of a lesion. Failure to follow these principles will frequently necessitate the removal of additional tissue, distortion of the specimen, or unnecessary damage to your patient.

GENERAL RULES

Size:
- If the lesion is small, less than 1 cm, it may be totally removed by an **excisional biopsy.**
- **If the lesion is larger than 1 cm, incisional biopsy(ies)** is/are performed.

Appearance:
- Choose the most suspicious area or areas, including the growing border of the lesion and some normal tissue. Collect several specimens when necessary.

Adequate section:
- With suture or pin, mark the location or orientation of the biopsy specimen and put it in the formalin immediately after it is removed from the patient. **DO NOT WAIT!!**

Anesthesia:
- When possible, use a block anesthesia rather than infiltration anesthesia which may distort the microscopic anatomy.

Anatomical considerations:
- When doing a biopsy, keep the incision within the long axis of major nerves and blood vessels.
- Attempt to keep all incision lines within the long axis of muscle tension to decrease dehiscence and scarring.

Cryosurgery or electrosurgery may be used by a trained person. However, there is greater risk of damaging the specimen and distorting the histology, causing difficulty in interpretation by your pathologist.

NOTE: ALL TISSUE REMOVED FROM THE BODY SHOULD BE SENT FOR PATHOLOGIC DIAGNOSIS. The above is a statement of the Joint Commission of Accreditation of Hospitals and all accredited hospitals abide by it. This is by far the safest and best practice to follow.

You may occasionally remove an extensive amount of tissue during gingivectomy or multiple extractions. Special arrangements with the local oral or medical pathologist can usually be made to have this extensive amount of periodontal and/or periapical tissue examined at a reasonable cost to your patient.

Six general rules for surgical removal of tissue have been discussed. State the major idea behind each key word.

Size: ______________________________

____

Appearance: ______________________________

____

Adequate section: ____________________

Location: ____________________

Anesthesia: ____________________

Anatomical considerations: ____________________

What should be done with all tissue removed from your patients? ____________________

General Surgical Techniques for Tissue Removal (Biopsy)

- **Excisional or Total Biopsy** is the removal of the entire lesion with an appropriate amount of normal marginal tissue. This technique is indicated for lesions less than one centimeter (<1.0 cm or <10 mm) in the greatest dimension. The usual margin of normal tissue is 2.0 mm beyond the clinical margin of the lesion. (See site selection for variations.)

  Plate IV, Fig. 85-89 illustrates an excisional biopsy of a benign hyperkeratotic lesion on the right buccal mucosa of a 59-year-old male.

- **Incisional or Wedge Biopsy** is the removal of a portion of a lesion. This technique is indicated for lesions greater than one centimeter (>1.0 cm or >10 mm) in their greatest dimension. You may desire to sample more than one site in large lesions by this technique.

  Plate II, Fig. 34-39 illustrates an incisional biopsy for a large soft tissue lesion on the maxillary labial gingivae.

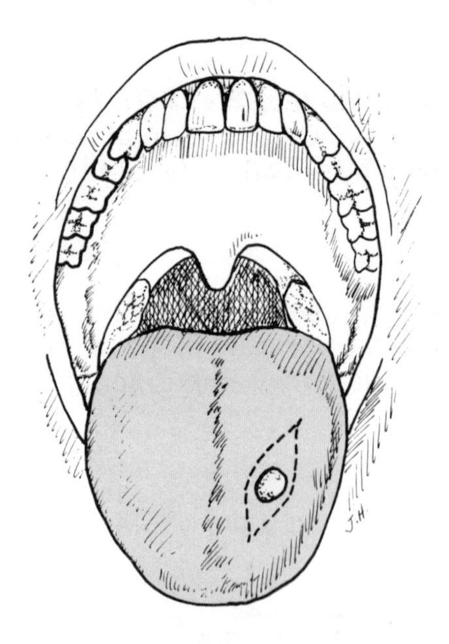

Figure II-1. Excisional biopsy is removal of the entire lesion

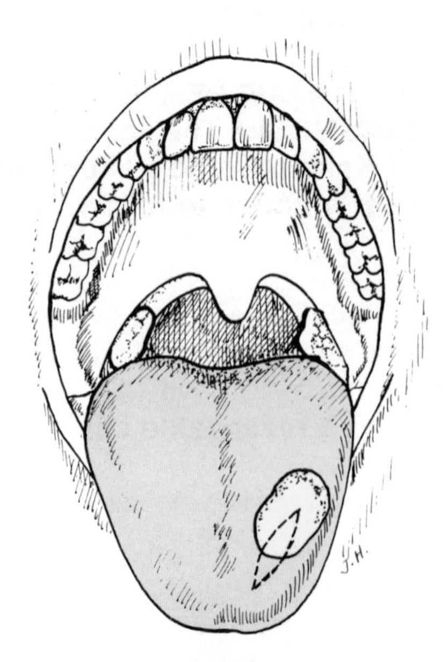

Figure II-2. Incisional biopsy is a removal of a representative sample of the lesion.

- **Bone or Open Biopsy** is the surgical incision, exposure, and removal of a representative piece of bone and/or soft tissue from a lesion in the bone. The bone biopsy may be incisional or excisional.

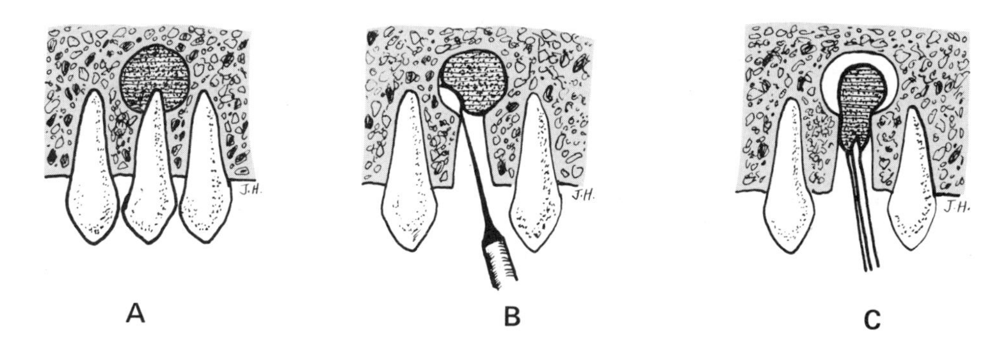

Figure II-3. Bone or Open Biopsy. A. Tooth with lesion at apex. B. After tooth extraction you can remove tissue through the extraction site. First, using a curette, loosen any attachment of the specimen to the bone. C. After you have curetted around the bony margin to loosen the specimen, you can grasp the specimen with tissue forceps. If the tooth is to be retained, tissue can be removed through an osseous window created in the bone (i.e., apioectomy).

NOTE: **Before an entry into a radiolucent bone lesion, a needle aspiration is strongly advised to rule out a vascular lesion. The presence of bright red blood under pressure would signify a vascular lesion within the bone. Incision into a vascular lesion in soft tissue or bone could have fatal results for your patient.**

- **Aspiration or Needle Biopsy** is the removal of a specimen by aspiration through a needle or trocar that is pierced through the skin or external surface of an organ and into the underlying tissue to be examined. (Used in dentistry primarily for a visual and/or biochemical analysis of cystic fluid, or fluid from a radiolucent bone lesion.)

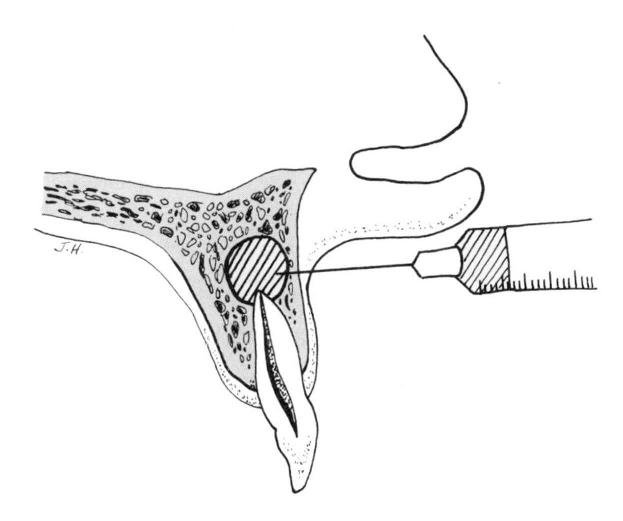

Figure II-4. Aspiration or Needle Biopsy

- **Punch Biopsy** is a method by which a small cylindrical piece of tissue for biopsy is removed by means of a special instrument that may penetrate into an organ or the skin. (Rarely used in oral lesions because of the ease of access with the scalpel.)

- **Exfoliate Cytology** is an examination of prepared desquamated cells to obtain a diagnosis. (This technique is not advocated except in rare instances of known irradiated cancer follow-up because of the ease of access and greater accuracy of scalpel biopsy.)

- **Curettage** is the removal of tissue by curettement which may be incisional or excisional in extent. The tissue is usually fragmented as in the surgical removal of a periapical lesion. (See **Figure II-3** on page 31.)

You have detected a 7 mm lesion on the tip of the tongue of one of your patients. You will probably use an ____________________ biopsy for this situation. If the lesion were 15 mm, would your choice be the same? ____________ (Yes/No) What method would you use now? ____________________ In either case, what must you include in your specimen along with lesion tissue? ____________________

What is a bone or open biopsy? ____________________

____

What essential precaution should be taken before incising into a radiolucent lesion in the jaws? ____________________

____

Describe the signs that would cause you to suspect an underlying vascular lesion. ______

____

Should you proceed with the biopsy? ____________ *(Yes/No) Why?* ____________

____

What is an aspiration or needle biopsy? ____________________

____

____

When is it used in dentistry? ____________________

____

What is a punch biopsy? ____________________

____

Is it used much in dentistry? ____________ *Why?* ____________________

Why is exfoliate cytology not used too often in dentistry? ____________________

____

Are there definite indications for its use? ____________ *When?* ____________

Biopsy by curettage usually results in tissue samples that are ____________________ *as in the removal of a periapical lesion.*

PERFORMING A SOFT TISSUE BIOPSY

Instruments:

- Retractor
- Scalpel (#15 blade)
- Fine tissue forceps or traction hook (Addision's tissue for cysts)
- Small straight pin
- Biopsy bottle containing 10% formalin (ten times the volume of the specimen, or more)
- Suture, needle holder, tissue scissors

Technique

Block anesthesia is obtained when possible and the tissue is immobilized with forceps, traction hook, or fine sutures.

Both incisions are eliptical, tapered and V-shaped.

The lesion is severed from its attachment with tissue scissors or scalpel. **Always put the specimen immediately in 10% formalin.** (Remember to gently blot the excess blood off the specimen with gauze. A cotton swab makes a good conveyor of the tissue specimen to the formalin bottle and prevents instrument contamination.)

Hemostatis is established and the wound edges are closed with interrupted sutures at intervals of 2-4 mm. Place six to eight sutures in all mobile tissue such as cheek or tongue. (If the biopsy is of the hard palate, the defect is usually covered with absorbable, oxidized cellulose, since complete closure may be impossible.)

The surgical technique for soft tissue biopsy involves the following basic four steps. Describe how each step should be completed and the instruments you should use for each step.

a. Anesthesia: ______________________________

____

b. Incision: ______________________________

____

c. Care of specimen: ______________________________

____

d. Hemostasis and closure: ______________________________

____

____

PERFORMING A HARD TISSUE (BONE) BIOPSY (FOR A RADIOLUCENT LESION)

Instruments:

Same as those for soft tissue biopsy, with the addition of
- Bur or chisel and mallet
- Curette

Technique

Anesthesia is obtained. **Aspirate the lesion with a 20-ga. needle.** If no bright red blood is aspirated, proceed.

Incise and reflect an adequate flap, either horizontal or vertical (one tooth anterior, including the papilla and obliquely forward). The flap margin should be **at least 2 mm and preferably 5 mm beyond your anticipated bony margins.** This will facilitate closure and healing by primary intention.

A circular piece of bone (window) is removed with either a bur or chisel from the external cortex to expose the lesion. A generous amount of tissue is carefully enucleated or curetted from the lesion and immediately placed in formalin.

Hemostasis is established, the flap reapposed, and the wound is closed.

Be sure to indicate to your pathologist that **both** soft tissue and bone are included.

Inform your patient that the report may take up to two weeks because of special handling required for the bone specimen.

STUDY EXERCISES—Hard Tissue Biopsy

1. *Following anesthesia, what essential procedure should be done before surgery is initiated to biopsy a lesion in bone?* ______________________________
____

2. *Enumerate the steps in performing a hard tissue biopsy and how the instruments are used.*

STEPS	*INSTRUMENTS*
a. ______________________	______________________
______________________	______________________
b. ______________________	______________________
______________________	______________________
c. ______________________	______________________
______________________	______________________
d. ______________________	______________________
______________________	______________________

e. ______________________ ______________________

______________________ ______________________

f. ______________________ ______________________

______________________ ______________________

STUDY EXERCISES—Hard Tissue Biopsy, Answers

1. *You **must** aspirate contents of lesion within bone before you begin surgery. Failure to do this may result in exposure of an aneurismic bone cyst and create a life-threatening bleeding problem for your patient.*

2. *a. Anesthesia is obtained and then aspirate lesion with a 20-ga. needle.*
   b. Incise and reflect mucoperiosteal flap with #15 blade in scalpel and periosteal elevator. Flap should provide at least 2 mm and preferably 5 mm bony margin.
   c. Remove circular piece of bone with bur or chisel and curette lesion contents—place into 10% formalin.
   d. Hemostasis and close flap with 3-0 silk suture.
   e. Indicate to your pathologist that both soft and hard tissue are included.
   f. Inform your patient that up to two weeks may be required because of special handling required for the bone specimen.

SITE SELECTION AND SURGICAL MODIFICATIONS

General Principles

The total amount of tissue removed in obtaining a surgical specimen will be influenced by:

- **The size of the lesion.**
- **The physical properties of the tissue.**
- **The malignant potential.**

Whatever the technique (incisional or excisional), it is necessary for you to include an adequate margin of normal tissue in your specimen. Your pathologist needs an adequate margin of normal tissue to compare the relationship between the normal and abnormal tissue. We will provide specific guidelines for the amount of surgical extension beyond the lesion or modifications in surgical technique in each of the subsequent sections.

The first and primary reason for removing a tissue specimen is to remove the entire lesion or a representative sample of the lesion plus an adequate normal border. This surgery should be done with the least amount of damage to oral structures.

General Rules:

- **Strive for an elliptical wedge of tissue. The surgical site is easier to suture closed.**

- **Incise parallel, not perpendicular, to nerves, arteries, and veins.**

- **Incise parallel, not perpendicular, to muscle fibers and attachments.**

- **If you have a choice, follow the line of stress or tension to minimize visibility of the scar (especially if extending onto vermillion border or lips).**

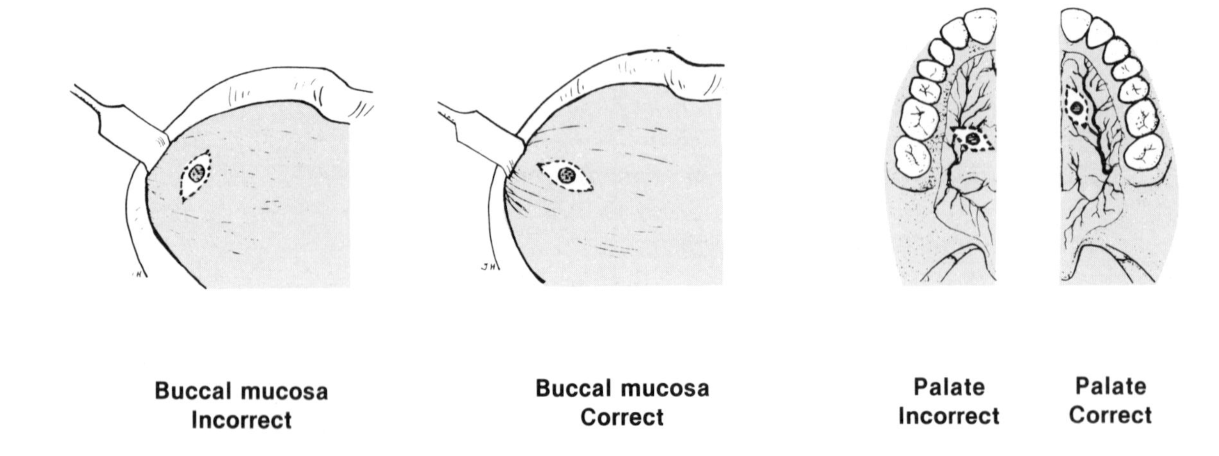

Figure II-5. Correct and Incorrect Application of General Rules for Biopsy Site Selection

Look at the following sketches of site selection. State whether the outline follows the general rules.

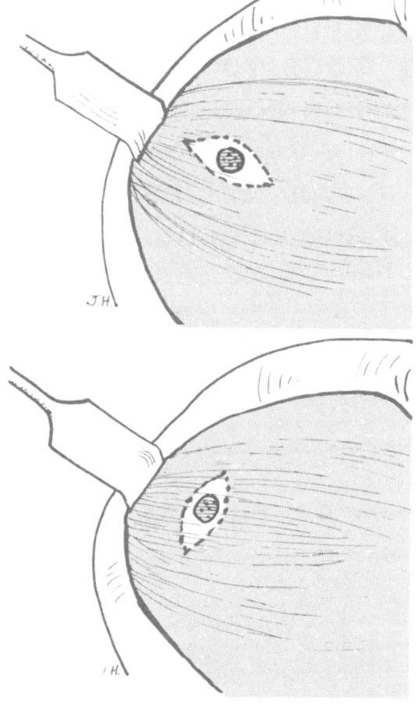

1. *Correct ______ Yes ______ No*
   *Why?*____

2. *Correct ______ Yes ______ No*
   *Why?*____

3. *Correct ______ Yes ______No*
   *Why?*____

4. *Correct ______ Yes ______ No*
   *Why?*____

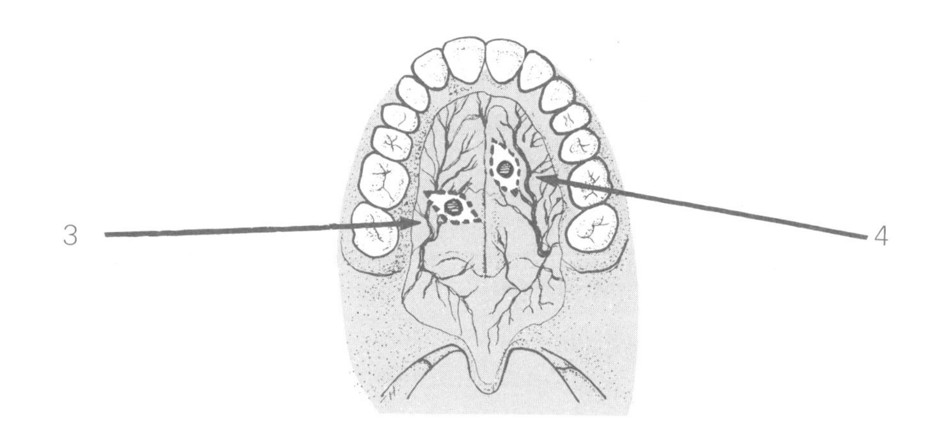

Excisional Biopsy

Usual Outline

The excisional technique, as discussed earlier, is used most often for lesions 1.0 cm (10 mm) or less in size. When making an elliptical incision on both sides of the lesion with your #15 Bard Parker scalpel blade, you will usually find that your incision will be about 5 mm beyond the lesion borders at either end, and usually about 2 mm from the lesion margin on the sides. The illustrations below show the usual outline for benign, non-invasive type lesions. The long axis of the incisions should follow the general rule for site selection.

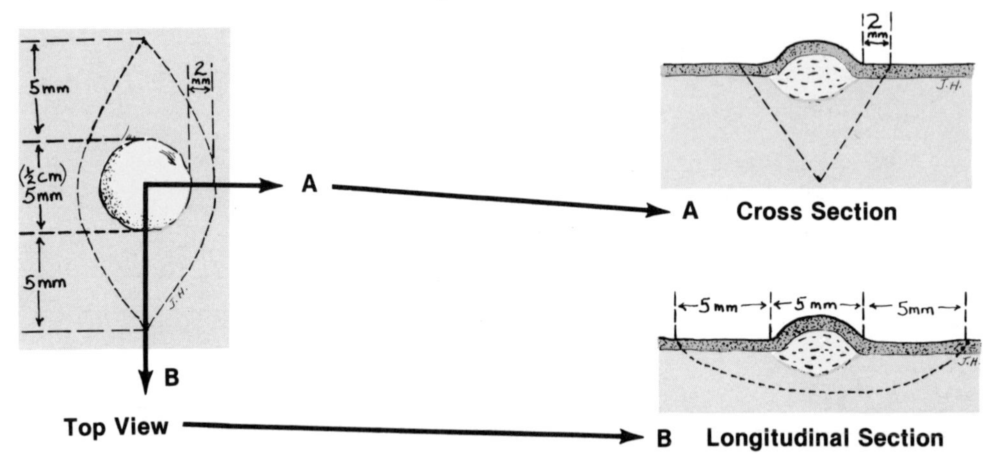

Figure II-6. Usual Outline Dimensions for a "Typical" Excisional Biopsy.

Surgical Modifications

Extension of Normal Tissue Borders

In most cases, excisional biopsy procedures require little modification of technique when dealing with different types of lesions. Modifications which may be required include:

Extending your surgical margins **at least 5 mm beyond the clinical margin** of the lesion. This is done for:

- Any pigmented lesions.
- Small vascular lesions (hemangiomas, lymphangiomas, angiokeratomas).
- Any small, rapidly growing, possibly malignant lesion.
- Lesions with diffuse borders.

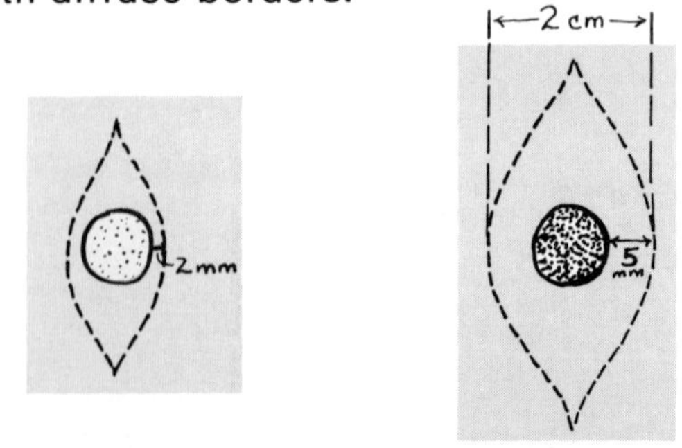

Figure II-7. Enlargement of Usual Excisional Biopsy Outline for Specific Lesions.

You can palpate the extension of the lesion below the clinical margin of the tissue in well-circumscribed and well-defined benign tumors. It will be necessary for you to modify your normal wedge biopsy technique so that the lateral surgical margins are more parallel and the base is wedge shaped to ensure that all the lesional tissue is removed (**Figure II-8B** below). This technique will help prevent recurrence of benign tumors removed by excisional biopsy. When this technique is used, you will need to deep suture the recessed wedge portion first, then close the more superficial portion (**Figure II-8C** below). This is usually a more complex procedure (see Unit III).

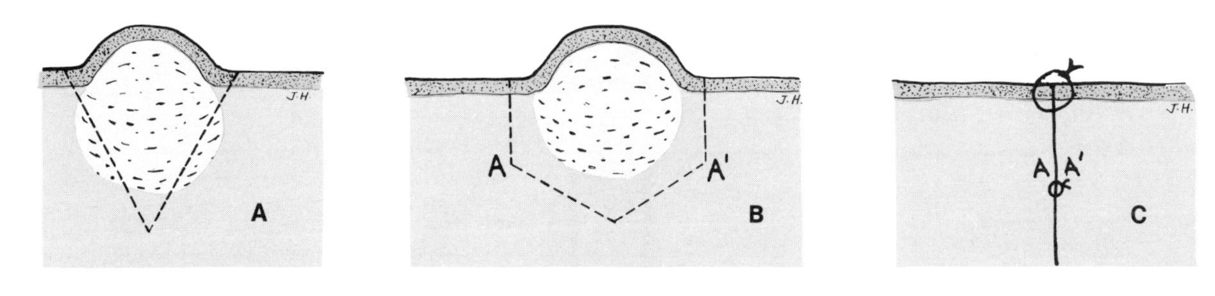

Figure II-8

Your ability to surgically close the modified outline as described above will depend upon the mobility of the particular tissue involved. This technique is generally used when sufficient soft tissue remains below the wound.

If you remove a block of tissue with a wide flat base (**Figure II-9B** below) closure will be difficult. If you are unable to close the base of the lesion, the wound will heal by primary intention at the outer margin, but will develop a hematoma internally (**Figure II-9C** below). The hematoma will require considerably longer to organize. It is also possible that oral flora trapped inside the void area could develop local infection with no source of drainage.

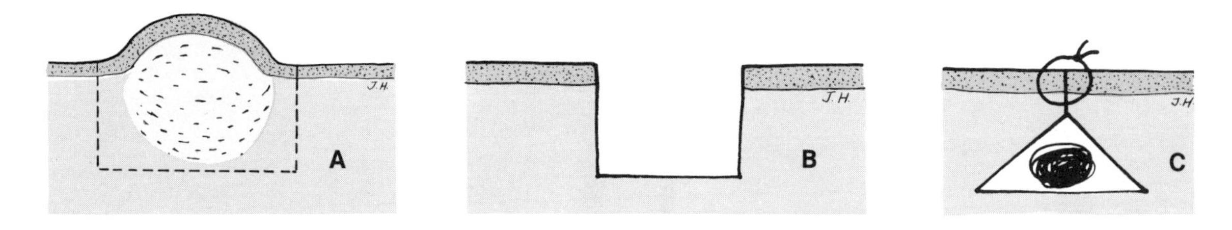

Figure II-9.

If you must remove a block of tissue from the palate or attached gingiva, especially if this tissue specimen is larger than 3 mm, you would best leave the wound "open" and cover it with a protective dressing. Remember, your ability to close your incision is related to the mobility of the underlying tissue.

Describe the characteristics of a "normal" excisional biopsy specimen. (Assume your lesion is 10 mm (1.0 cm) in diameter.)

Length of incision: ____________________

Width of incision: ____________________

Depth of incision: ____________________

Describe the two main modifications for excisional biopsy and the indications for these modifications.

Extending ____________________
When used? ____________________
Why? ____________________

Modify surgical ____________ *by* ____________
When used? ____________________
Why is this done? ____________________

If you feel the normal wedge-shaped specimen would not include the deeper margins of a benign tumor, when would you consider the modified wedge as described on page 39?
____

If the lesion were on your patient's hard palate, would you also follow this technique?
______ *Yes* ______ *No. Why?* ____________________

What would be the reasons for not incising a "flat floor" to the specimen? ____________________

Incisional Biopsy

In lesions requiring incisional biopsy techniques, it is necessary to sample the area or areas of the lesion that will provide the most histopathologic information leading to the diagnosis of the lesion.

The usual incisional biopsy is an eliptical wedge of tissue removed from **a portion of the lesion.** After you have considered the general rules of site selection, your incisional technique should result in a tissue specimen that contains a deep, thin sample of the lesion, plus an adequate margin of normal tissue.

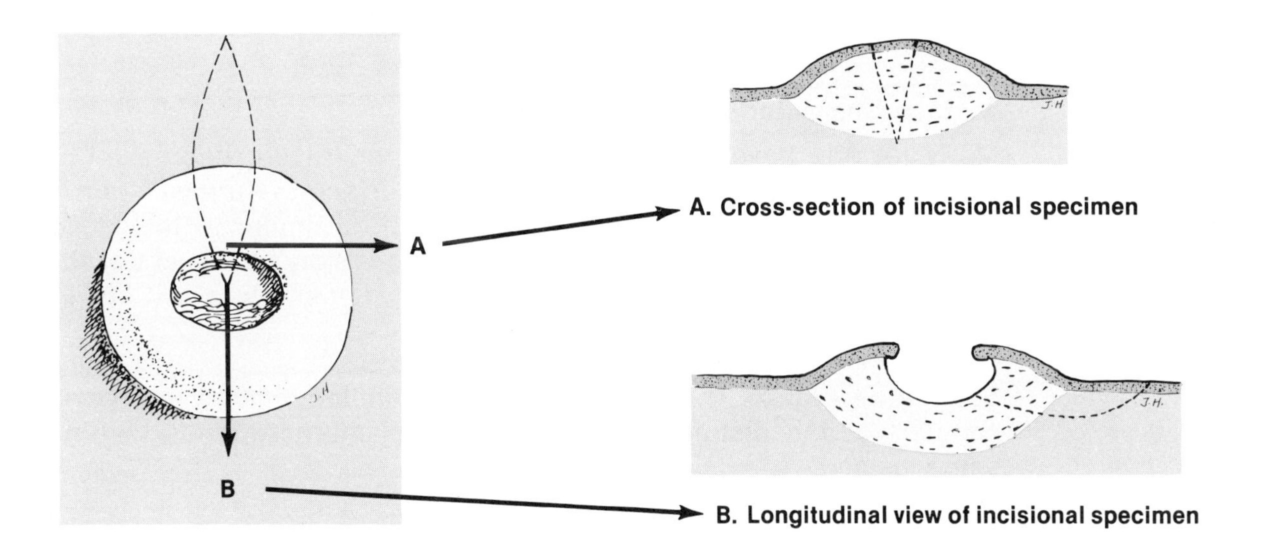

Figure II-10. Usual outline for an incisional tissue specimen. Dimensions are not specified because these lesions can range in sizes greater than 1.0 cm.

NOTE: IN LESIONS WITH AREAS OF ULCERATIONS, IT IS ESSENTIAL THAT YOU INCLUDE A SMALL PORTION OF THE ULCERATION AS WELL AS A REPRESENTATIVE SECTION OF THE INTACT LESION (NEAR THE PERIPHERY OF THE ULCER) WITH ADJACENT NORMAL TISSUE. (See Figure II-10 above.)

Physical Properties Influencing Site Selection

Factors in this section are discussed individually; however, most lesions show combinations of these properties.

- **Definition of Margins**

  Lesions that have irregular or indistinct margins will require you to extend the surgical margin **to at least 5 mm beyond the apparent clinical margin of the lesion.** This surgical extension ensures an adequate margin of normal tissue. The more indistinct the lesion, the wider the border of normal tissue you should include. See **Figure II-11**, page 42.

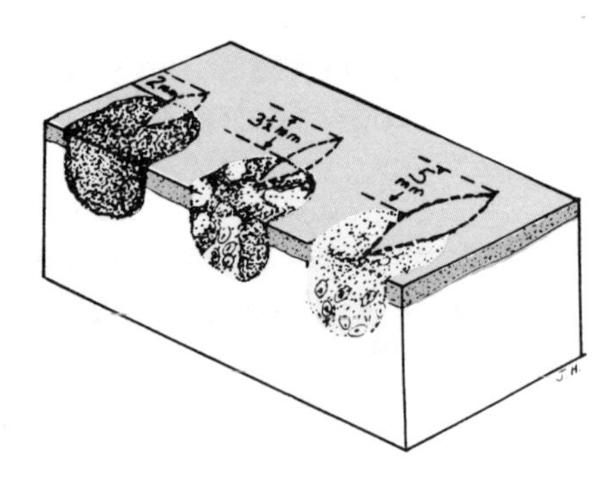

Figure II-11. Definition of margins.

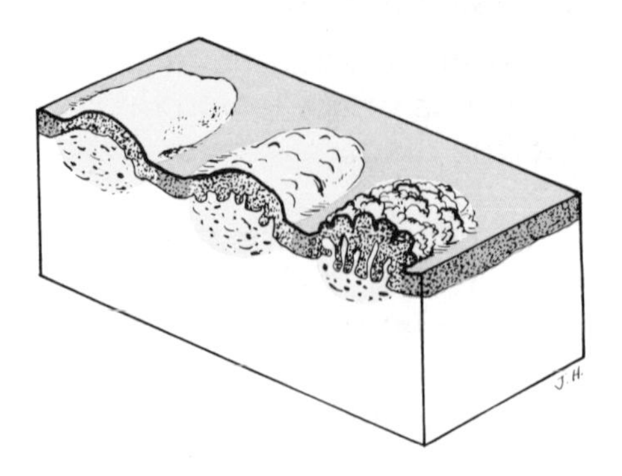

Figure II-12. Surface Texture

- **Surface Characteristics**

  Many lesions have irregular surfaces, either raised, depressed, or a combination of both. In some lesions, the surface texture will be rough. In other lesions the surface will be smooth or similar to the adjacent normal tissue. It is necessary to survey the lesion and select a site or sites which most adequately represent the lesion as a whole. (See **Figure II-12** above.)

  See **Plate I, Fig. 25.** This lesion should be sampled in more than one site because of the distinctly different surface characteristics within the same lesion.

- **Depth of Extension**

  Some lesions extend deep into the subjacent anatomic structures (i.e., fat, skeletal muscle, bone). These lesions require that you remove a deeper tissue specimen than with your normal surgical technique. **As long as vital structures are not compromised, it is better to extend the depth of your surgical incision to ensure you have normal tissue below.**

  However, in large lesions that may grossly involve vital anatomical structures, you may need only to sample to the normal depth to determine a diagnosis for future surgery.

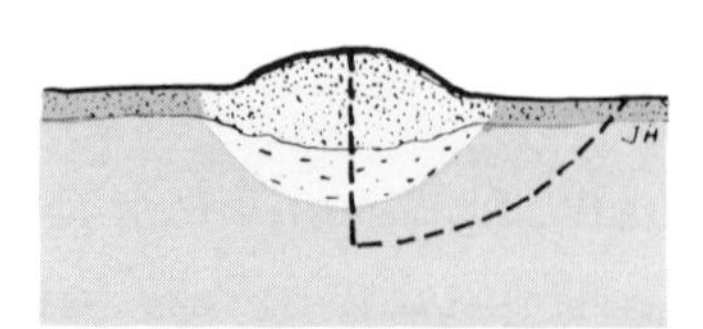

A. Usual incisional biopsy.

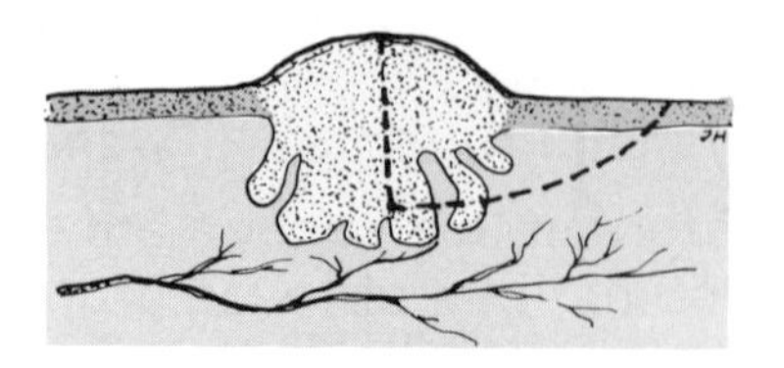

B. Modified.

Figure II-13. Modification of depth for incisional biopsy to prevent damage to underlying anatomical structures. A. Usual incisional biopsy. B. Modified outline to avoid a nerve.

In biopsying soft tissue lesions that extend down to but do not involve the periosteum, you will need to extend your surgical incision **to include the periosteum.**

- **Quality of Tissue**

Some lesions are necrotic, friable, errosive, or bullous-vesicular in nature. These lesions require special attention to surgical outline and handling technique due to an undermining of normal tissue.

In selecting the surgical site, **it is necessary for you to extend your surgical margin at least 3 mm beyond your normal 2 mm margin so that your margin is now at least 5 mm beyond the clinical margin of the lesion.**

This is especially true when the margin of the ulcer is within 1 mm of the margin of erythema or for those ulcerated lesions in which the ulcer comprises more than 50% of the lesion. (See Evaluation of Degree of Difficulty, Unit III.)

Lesions which involve a separation at or near the basal layer of epithelium usually extend further under normal tissue histologically than is clinically apparent.

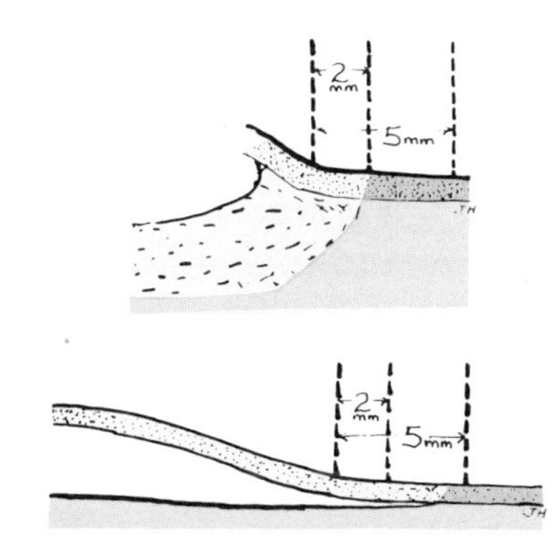

Figure II-14. For necrotic, friable, errosive, or bullous-vesicular lesions, extension of surgical margin must include adequate normal tissue.

In these types of lesions, the integrity of the apparently normal tissue is usually compromised so that special care in handling the tissue during surgery is mandatory.

Specific Example

In **bullous-vesicular lesions**, over-aggressive handling of the delicate tissue can cause additional separation of the epithelium (Nikolsky's sign). If the epithelium completely separates from the underlying connective tissue, histopathologic interpretation is seriously impaired.

- **Pigmentation and Vascularity**

NOTE: Pigmented or vascular lesions SHOULD NEVER BE BIOPSIED BY INCISIONAL TECHNIQUES.

There currently exists controversy over the use of incisional biopsies for pigmented lesions such as nevi, ephilids, lentigenes. The possibility of stimulating benign lesions to become malignant or the seeding of a malignant lesion have been cited in the literature and has generated much debate. It would therefore be wise for you, as a general practitioner, to refer large pigmented lesions to a specialist.

In the case of vascular lesions, the possibility of creating life-threatening hemorrhage is significant. These conditions must also be treated by a specialist.

- **Soft Tissue or Bone**

  Whether the lesion is in soft tissue or bone will influence your site selection. Radiolucent bony lesions require that you first aspirate the lesion, then reflect a periosteal flap to gain access. The specific flap outline should follow the rules for flaps discussed elsewhere.

- **Growth Rate**

  In some benign tumors, growth rate may vary.

  In lesions that are clinically benign, the area showing the most rapid growth should be biopsied.

  If you have a slow-growing area, you usually have a well-circumscribed lesion and need only a 2 mm margin.

  If you have a rapidly growing tumor, you should extend your margin to 5 mm.

STUDY EXERCISES—Modifications for Incisional Biopsy Procedure

1. *For the following schematic diagram of a lesion requiring the removal of a tissue specimen, draw the ideal outline for your incisions and give quantitative measurements of your desired extensions beyond the lesion for each view.*

   a. *This 15 mm (1.5 cm) lesion on the palate just to the midline, appears to be superficial in nature with very little invasion into underlying tissue. It is well away from any "important" anatomical structures. Borders are well defined.*

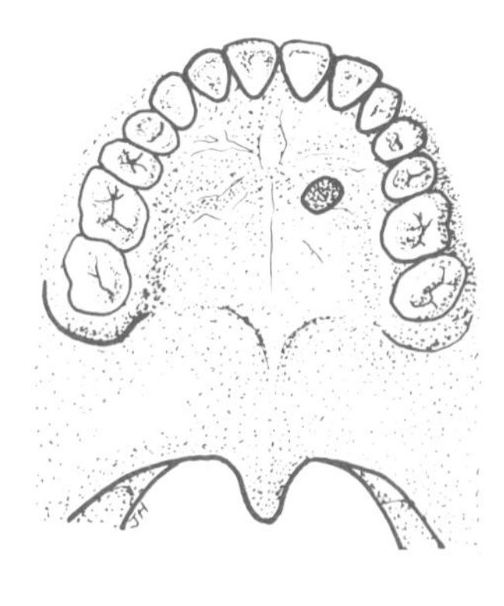

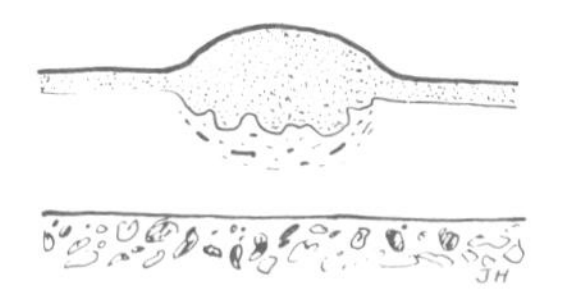

Longitudinal View

Extension into normal tissue = ______ mm beyond clinical margin

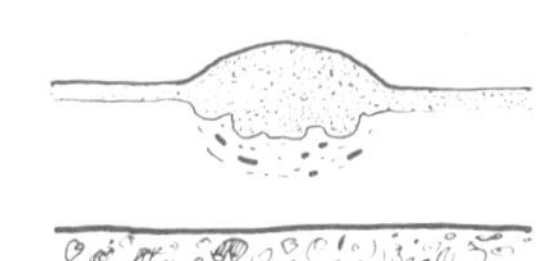

Cross-section View

Extension into normal tissue = ______ mm below lesion

   b. *If the above lesion was located instead on the lateral aspect of the palate directly over your greater palatine artery and nerve, would you use the same outline and depth for your incisions? ______ (Yes/No). Explain: ______________________*

____

____

1. c. *What if you thought the lesion in question (1a) extended deeper into the tissue? What would determine the depth of your incision?* ______________________

____

____

____

d. *What if the lesion appeared to be very large (30 mm) and deep? How would you modify your surgical outline?*
*Longitudinally:*______________________________________

____

Cross Sectionally: ______________________________________

____

STUDY EXERCISES—*Answers*

1. a.

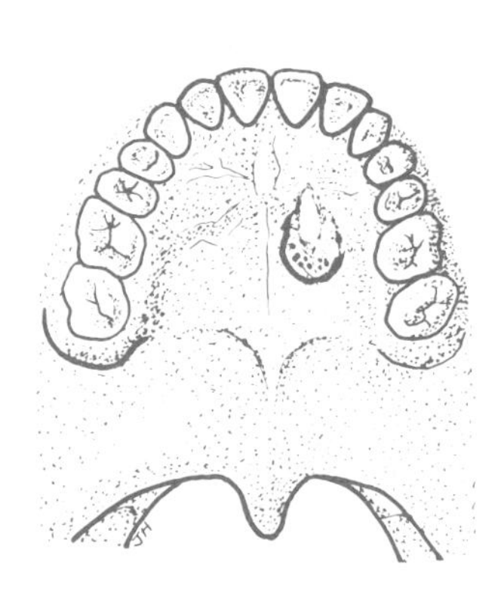

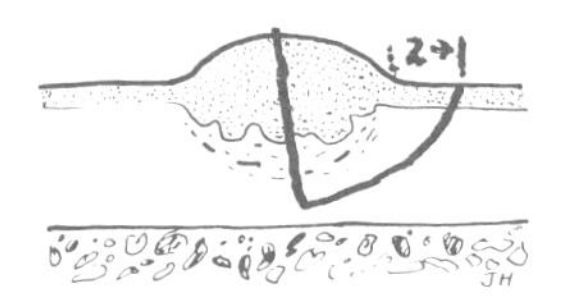

Extension into normal tissue = 2 mm beyond clinical margin

Longitudinal View

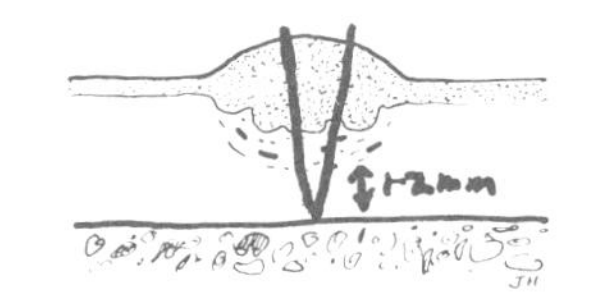

Extension into normal tissue = 1-2 mm below lesion

Cross-section View

b. *Yes. You should be sure you are parallel to the underlying nerves, arteries and veins.*

c. *The depth of your incision should be adjusted, depending upon the proximity to important anatomical structures (nerves, arteries, and veins). If you consider the lesion to extend into the palatal bone, you would be correct to remove a superficial portion for microscopic examination concurrent with referral.*

d. *As with "c" above, you should consider referral at this time and possibly remove a small specimen for microscopic examination.*

STUDY EXERCISES—Clinical Case Simulations

Look at each of the following clinical cases. Evaluate each of the eight physical properties and check those properties that would cause you to modify the basic incisional surgical procedure. State the modification that would be necessary. Some may require no modification.

Physical Properties Requiring Alteration of Basic Surgical Technique

Lesion	*Definition of Margins*	*Surface Characteristics*	*Depth of Extension*	*Quality of Tissue*	*Pigmentation*	*Vascularity*	*Soft Tissue or Bone*	*Growth Rate*	*Surgical Modifications Required*
1. Fig. 34 This is a well circumscribed superficial lesion of at least 1 year's duration.	☐	☐	☐	☐	☐	☐	☐	☐	________
2. Fig. 65 This pigmented lesion is superficial. It has been present for 10 years.	☐	☐	☐	☐	☐	☐	☐	☐	________
3. Fig. 19 This lesion in the floor of the mouth has been present for one month. It is slightly indurated on palpation.	☐	☐	☐	☐	☐	☐	☐	☐	________
4. Fig. 25 This lesion on the alveolar ridge has an irregular surface that becomes exophytic on the mesial aspect. It has been present for three months. The lesion appears to involve the underlying bone.	☐	☐	☐	☐	☐	☐	☐	☐	________
5. Fig. 57 This red lesion has been there as long as the patient can remember. Periapical radiographs of this area show multilocular lesions in the bone.	☐	☐	☐	☐	☐	☐	☐	☐	________
6. Fig. 47 This lesion has persisted for two months, despite your attempts at conservative therapy. Upon palpation, you find the lesion extending into the body of the tongue.	☐	☐	☐	☐	☐	☐	☐	☐	________
7. Fig. 55 This slightly irregular, well delineated white lesion has been present for 2 months and has not changed size.	☐	☐	☐	☐	☐	☐	☐	☐	________
8. Fig. 70 This white lesion on the floor of the mouth has an unknown duration. It is all superficial in nature.	☐	☐	☐	☐	☐	☐	☐	☐	________

STUDY EXERCISES—Answers

Physical Properties Requiring Alteration of Basic Surgical Technique

Lesion	*Definition of Margins*	*Surface Characteristics*	*Depth of Extension*	*Quality of Tissue*	*Pigmentation*	*Vascularity*	*Soft Tissue or Bone*	*Growth Rate*	*Surgical Modifications Required*
1. Fig. 34									None required.
2. Fig. 65	X				X		S		Extend specimen margin at least 5 mm beyond clinical margin.
3. Fig. 19			X				S	X	Because of induration, surgical incisions should be extended deeper to include a normal border below the lesion.
4. Fig. 25		X	X				b		The irregular surface of this lesion would require you to take at least 2 specimens. The depth of the biopsy should also be increased due to the bony involvement.
5. Fig. 57	X	X	X			X	S b		You should never do incisional biopsies on vascular lesions.
6. Fig. 47	X	X	X	X					Extend normal margins at least 5 mm beyond clinical margin and depth should go below the lesion.
7. Fig. 55							S		No modifications necessary.
8. Fig. 70							S		No modifications of surgical technique are needed, but you would be wise to take multiple samples.

NOTE: These study exercises were intended to give you experience in modifying your planned surgical outline depending upon the characteristics of the lesion. You will have additional use for the physical characteristics of lesions when assessing the relative degree of difficulty of each surgical biopsy.

- **Malignant Potential**

When biopsying lesions that have a potential for malignancy, it is necessary for you to look for and sample the areas of the lesion that are the most suspicious. The most positive sites will usually show some or all of the following characteristics.

1. Induration (hard, firm)
2. Fixed to underlying tissue
3. Fissuring or cracking
4. Friable tissue that bleeds easily
5. Area of rapid growth
6. Recurrent or persistent lesion
7. Erythema (redness)

STUDY EXERCISES—Malignant Potential

1. When you look at and/or palpate a lesion, what clues would cause you to suspect you were involved with a malignant lesion? (Especially viewing the lesion over a period of time.)

a. ______________ *e.* ______________
b. ______________ *f.* ______________
c. ______________ *g.* ______________
d. ______________

2. From palpation of the lesion, what information would suggest "malignancy" to you?

a. ______________
b. ______________

3. Can you ever expect to see a malignant condition that does not show any of the above characteristics? ______ *Yes* ______ *No. Why?* ______________

____

4. Would the presence of any of the above characteristics automatically imply malignancy? ______ *Yes* ______ *No. Why?* ______________

____

STUDY EXERCISES—Malignant Potential, Answers

1. See page 48.
2. See page 48.
3. Yes. Malignant lesions in their early stages may not have developed to the level necessary to show these signs, i.e., early white lesions must be examined microscopically to determine if they are malignant.
4. No. Malignancy is a histopathological condition and must be determined by microscopic study. Other conditions may show some of the signs and not be neoplastic, i.e., pyogenic granuloma.

CARE AND HANDLING OF THE SPECIMEN FOLLOWING SURGERY

You surgically remove tissue to provide a sample for your pathologist to examine. Improper handling of tissue during and after surgery can cause irreversible damage. Damaged specimens cannot be adequately interpreted by your pathologist and can, therefore, reduce your ability to manage your patient's problem. **Always follow these precautions to avoid damaging the specimen:**

1. Gently blot excess blood off the specimen with a gauze sponge.

2. Orientation may be enhanced by placing a suture or a straight pin to denote the epithelium or direction of the lesion (i.e., anterior, posterior, etc.), taking care not to distort the histology of the lesion with the suture.

3. Place specimen into formalin without delay.

4. A cotton swab or gauze makes a good conveyor of the tissue specimen to the formalin bottle and prevents instrument contamination. Sometimes a thin flat biopsy (i.e., from the floor of the mouth) may be placed flat on a section of thin cardboard to prevent folding.

5. Make sure the bottle contains 10% formalin in at least ten times the volume of the specimen.

6. As soon as the tissue is removed from its bed, place gauze packs over the biopsy site and attend to the specimen. Do not return to the patient until the tissue has been completely immersed in formalin. (Specimens may get lost. Dehydrated tissue may be difficult to interpret.)

7. Immediately after closing the wound, you should complete the laboratory request form to the pathologist. (See page 52.)

8. If multiple biopsies are taken, they should be placed in separate bottles and designated A, B, C, with appropriate sketches and a description of each.

9. If the bottle is to be mailed, a very careful sealing of the cap is absolutely essential to prevent leakage. The bottle is labeled in a simple manner, packaged carefully to prevent breakage, and sent to your pathologist.

10. If there is an especially urgent or strong suspicion of malignancy, a phone call to the pathologist is indicated.

11. Examples of inadequate tissue specimens.
    - Inadequate size (See Plate IV, Figure 108)
    - Inadequate depth (See Plate IV, Figures 105-107)
    - Inadequate margins (See Plate IV, Figures 109-112)

    In these tumor sections there is inadequate normal tissue at either the lateral or deep margins. Further surgery must be performed to completely remove the lesion.

12. Examples of tissue damage due to unacceptable handling techniques.
    - Tissue forcep marks (See Plate IV, Figures 102 and 103)
    - Stretch and crush artifacts (See Plate IV, Figure 104)
    - Periodontal plaque iatrogenically introduced into specimen (See Plate IV, Figure 101)

STUDY EXERCISES:

The care and handling of a tissue specimen following surgery is of extreme importance. In the spaces below write out the necessary steps for the care and handling of a tissue specimen.

1. *Following removal of tissue from mouth you should gently ______________ off the excess ______________ with a ______________ sponge.*

2. *Specimen should be ______________ by use of a ______________ or ______________ ______________ to denote the epithelium or ______________ of the lesion.*

3. *Place specimen into ______________ without ______________.*

4. *You may use a ______________ ______________ or ______________ to convey the tissue specimen to the formalin bottle.*

5. *Make sure the specimen bottle contains 10% ______________ in at least ______________ times the volume of the specimen.*

6. *Should you attend to the tissue or the surgical site first? ______________ Why? ______________*

7. *When should the laboratory report form be completed? ______________ ______________*

8. *How should you handle multiple specimens from the same lesion? ______________ ______________*

9. *What special precautions should you take if bottles are to be mailed? ______________ ______________ and ______________.*

10. *If you have a strong suspicion of malignancy you should ______________ your pathologist.*

COMPLETION OF THE REQUEST FOR LABORATORY STUDY FORM

The pathology request form should contain:

1. The patient's name, age, sex, race, office chart or hospital number, and address.
2. The surgeon's name, office, date of surgery, and signature.
3. Description of lesion: location, duration, size, shape, color, exophytic, endophytic, induration, fixation, fissuring, friability, hemorrhage, etc.
4. Sketch of the recognizable area of the lesion and biopsy site with sufficient labeling of anatomic structures.
5. Relevant medical history, past history, physical findings, symptoms, and radiographic findings.
6. Whether lymphadenopathy is present before biopsy.
7. A differential, clinical and/or tentative diagnosis of the biopsy.

Request for lab study is a medical-legal document and care should be exercised in the completion and the accuracy of the data presented. The patient's name and a signature by the practitioner are mandatory.

See page 52 for an example of a typical form.

NOTE: Pathology laboratories use a variety of request forms tailored to their specific needs. It is generally of great help to both dentist and pathologist to include standard sketches of the oral cavity from different perspectives on the printed request form. (Refer to example of printed sketches shown in Figure II-15 below.)

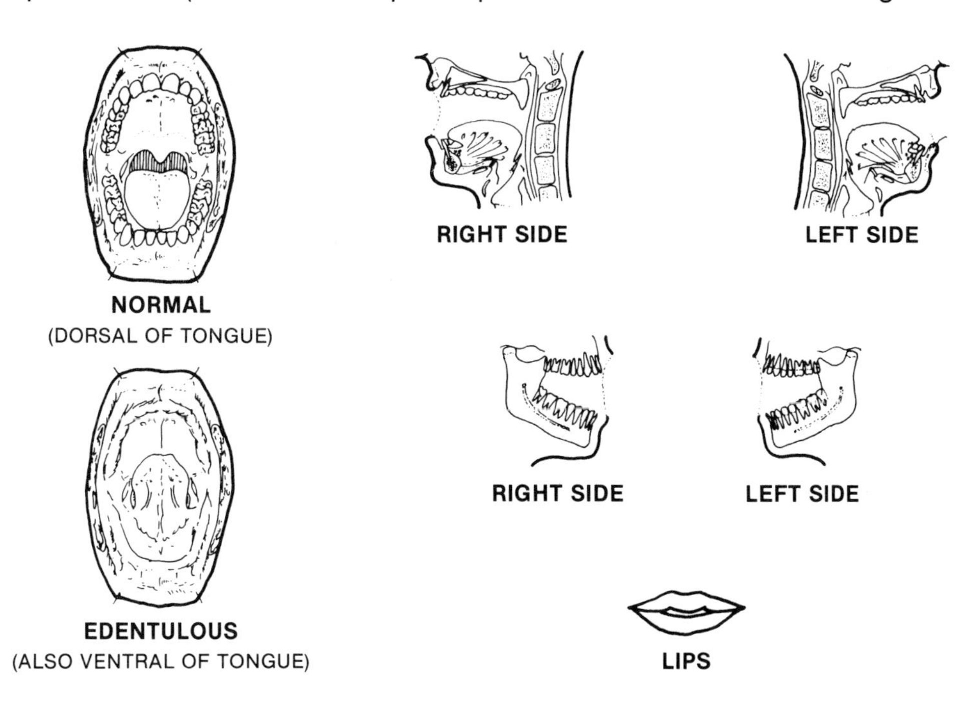

Figure II-15. Sample anatomical sketches used on laboratory request forms. (Courtesy of Albert F. Morgan, DDS.)

FOR LABORATORY USE ONLY

ACCESSION NO. ______

DATE RECEIVED ______

DATE DECAL ______

DECAL COMPLETED ______

REQUEST FOR LABORATORY STUDY

1 PATIENT'S NAME Mr. Alexander Swenson Age 72 Sex M Race W

2 PATIENT'S ADDRESS 1905 Boronna Ave

3 DOCTOR'S NAME Dr. Dennis J. Hansen Phone 555-1212

4 DOCTOR'S ADDRESS 395 Ridgemont Drive
NUMBER AND STREET

Seattle Washington 98105
CITY STATE ZIP CODE

5 DESCRIPTION OF LESION (INCLUDE LOCATION, DURATION, SIZE AND COLOR)

30 x 40 mm (3.0 x 4.0 cm) Raised, Indurated, White with red areas. Lesion has a central fissure located at the occlusal line (plane). Bleeds easily. lesion is on the right Buccal mucosa approaching the Right commissure

Sketch of Lesion Site

Rt. max cheek; mand cheek; specimen site; fissure

6 ASSOCIATED FINDINGS AND PAST HISTORY (INCLUDING PREVIOUS BIOPSY ACCESSION NO.)

Duration - Several months. Previously treated by a physician but has not resolved. Lymphadenopathy negative Before Surgery.

7 SYMPTOMS Painful to speak, masticate and touch.

8 RADIOGRAPHIC FINDINGS ◯ Radiographs Enclosed Negative

9 CLINICAL IMPRESSION Squamous Cell Carcinoma.

10 TYPE OF BIOPSY: ✓ Incisional ◯ Excisional ◯ Aspiration ◯ Curettage ◯ Other

11 Date tissue removed: 11/5/76 TIME: ☒ A.M. ☐ P.M. 12 Dennis J Hansen DDS
Doctor's Signature

REV. 11/75 1 75 2140

Given the following information, write out a request for laboratory study on the form provided on this page. Check your responses by comparing your answers with those on page 52.

1. *See Figure #8. A 72-year-old Caucasian male carpenter, presents your office for routine care. In your initial examination, you notice a 3.0 x 4.0 cm white lesion of the right commissure and cheek that is raised, roughened and fissured. It has been present for six to nine months. His physician has been painting the lesion, but it hasn't healed and it is painful when speaking or eating. No lymphadenopathy was found.*

   Your decision is to do a biopsy immediately to avoid additional delay. Please complete the request for laboratory study.

REQUEST FOR LABORATORY STUDY

1. **Patient's Name** **Age** **Sex** **Race**
2. **Patient's Address**
3. **Doctor's Name** **Phone**
4. **Doctor's Address**

   Number and Street

   City State Zip Code
5. **Description of Lesion** (Include location, duration, size and color)
6. **Sketch of Lesion Site**
7. **Associated Findings and Past History (including previous Biopsy Accession No.)**
8. **Symptoms**
9. **Radiographic Findings** ☐ **Radiographs Enclosed**
10. **Clinical Impression**

Type of Biopsy: ☐ **Incisional** ☐ **Excisional** ☐ **Aspiration** ☐ **Curettage** ☐ **Other**

12. **Date tissue removed:** **Time:** ☐ **A.M.** ☐ **P.M.**

13. Doctor's Signature

Compare your laboratory request form with the correct form on Page 52.

UNIT III

EVALUATION OF DEGREE OF DIFFICULTY AS A CRITERION FOR REFERRAL

Philosophy of Approach
The Factors
General Guideline

PRE-TEST UNIT III

- *Answer the following questions.*
- *Compare your answers with those below. If all responses are correct, proceed to Unit IV. If only some responses are correct, study Unit III.*

Questions

For each of the lesions below, state the overall degree of difficulty for biopsying.

Case:	*Degree of Difficulty* Easy → to → Difficult			
	0	*1*	*2*	*3*
1. See Figure 2	☐	☐	☐	☐
2. See Figure 24	☐	☐	☐	☐
3. See Figure 50	☐	☐	☐	☐
4. See Figure 57	☐	☐	☐	☐
5. See Figure 16	☐	☐	☐	☐

PRE-TEST—Answers

1)-0; 2)-3; 3)-2; 4)-3; 5)-3

CONTENT FOR UNIT III

EVALUATION OF DEGREE OF DIFFICULTY AS A CRITERION FOR REFERRAL

PHILOSOPHY OF APPROACH

As with most dental procedures, the level of special skills required to perform a biopsy may vary. The degree of difficulty for a specific biopsy situation is dependent on its location, size, type of lesion, malignant potential, and your patient's general health. It is our intent in this unit to teach you a technique to evaluate the degree of surgical difficulty for a particular lesion. It is not our intent to dictate specific criteria for referral to a specialist. Rather, it is our goal to enable you to properly evaluate each case and recognize potential problems that may be associated with an increase in degree of difficulty. You will then be able to make a decision to biopsy or refer after assessment of the clinical situation and your own surgical ability.

THE FACTORS

Once the decision has been made for biopsy, you must decide whether you should do the procedure or refer the case to someone with more skill in the required technique. The following factors can be used as a guideline for interpreting the degree of difficulty for each lesion. On the **"Key to Biopsy Evaluation Summary of Factors"** provided, we have made an assessment of the contributing difficulty component of each factor and developed a rating scale from 0 to 3. From analysis of factor ratings, plus your overall assessment of your patient and the specific situation involved, you can make a more informed decision. Ultimate evaluation of the degree of difficulty is dependent upon the inter-relationship of all factors. This will be discussed after you have developed the ability to identify and categorize the factors.

To help you put the whole biopsy process together, we have developed the one-page summary form shown on Page 56, "Evaluation and Treatment Record for Oral Lesions". This form should be useful in routine practice to assist you in properly managing oral lesions.

The factors which will be considered in more detail include:

- **Patient's general health**
- **Malignant potential of the lesion**
- **Physical properties of the lesion**
- **Size of the lesion**
- **Degree of surgical access**
- **Overall difficulty**

Evaluation and Treatment Record for Oral Lesions

Patient's Name ______________________

Address ______________________

____

Date lesion initially detected ______________

Initial Action Required:

☐ 1. Observe for 7-14 days
☐ 2. Non-surgical treatment
☐ 3. Request laboratory tests
☐ 4. Malignant potential high—biopsy now
☐ 5. Make decision to biopsy

Histologic Examination Required: ☐ Yes ☐ No

Method

☐ Incisional ☐ Bone
☐ Excisional ☐ Aspiration
☐ Other: ______________

Pre-Surgical Evaluation:

	0	1	2	3	Comments
1. Patient's general health	☐	☐	☐	☐	
2. Malignant potential	☐	☐	☐	☐	
3. Physical properties					
A. Definition of margins	☐	☐	☐		
B. Surface characteristics	☐	☐	☐		
C. Depth of extension	☐	☐	☐		
D. Quality of tissue	☐	☐	☐		
E. Pigmentation	☐	☐	☐	☐	
F. Vascularity	☐	☐	☐	☐	
G. Soft tissue or bone	☐	☐	☐	☐	
H. Growth rate	☐	☐	☐	☐	
I. Overall effect of physical properties	☐	☐	☐	☐	
4. Size of lesion	☐	☐	☐	☐	
5. Degree of surgical access					
A. Ability to see	☐	☐	☐	☐	
B. Ability to reach	☐	☐	☐	☐	
C. Ability to stabilize	☐	☐	☐	☐	
D. Underlying anatomy	☐	☐	☐	☐	
6. OVERALL DIFFICULTY	☐	☐	☐	☐	

Who Did Surgery?

☐ I did
☐ Referred to ______________________

____

Your Name ______________

Address ______________

Phone Number ______________

To Whom Was Specimen Submitted?

____

Date:

____

Pathologist's Report Received:

Date: ______________________

Comments:

☐ **Neoplastic**
- ☐ Benign
- ☐ Malignant
- ☐ Pre-malignant

☐ **Non-Neoplastic**
- ☐ Reactive
- ☐ Inflammatory
- ☐ Systemic

Course of Action

Referral to:

☐ Tumor board and oncologist:

____

☐ Oral surgeon:

____

☐ Physician:

____

My Treatment:

☐ Total removal
☐ Remove etiology
☐ Other: ______________________

Treatment Results: ______________________

____

____

Follow-Up Results: ______________________

____

____

____

Figure III-1. Evaluation and Treatment Record for Oral Lesions

1. Patient's General Health

An important factor in any medical procedure is your patient's general health. Complicating conditions in general health, which are not anticipated or managed, can turn an otherwise simple procedure into an acute emergency. Adequate pre-surgical review of the health history and thorough clinical examinations will be of great help in reducing the chance of an emergency.

The rating scale for difficulty has been divided into the following categories:

0—no history of medical problems or clinical conditions requiring modification in biopsy procedure.

1—history of medical problems which do not require a physician's consultation or modification of technique (i.e., drug allergies, some drug reactions, previous unrelated surgeries).

2—medical history reveals conditions requiring a physician's consultation but **no modification** in surgical technique (i.e., rheumatic fever).

3—medical history reveals conditions that require physician's consultation **and modification** of surgical technique (i.e., hemophilia, cardiovascular disease, etc.).

How would you rate the following cases as to the degree of difficulty presented by the patient's medical history.

Case #1—A 65-year-old patient presents with a 4 mm lesion in the anterior lateral border of the tongue. A review of the medical history reveals a history of childhood diseases, plus appendectomy 10 years ago. She has not had a physical exam for two years. She complains of polyurea and when you take her blood pressure, you obtain a 160/100 reading.
Rating ______

Case #2—A 35-year-old patient has a raised mass on the buccal mucosa associated with the linea alba. A review of the medical history is negative, except for a 20-year history of hay fever and allergy to "soaps."
Rating ______

Case #3—A 50-year-old man presents with a white lesion in the floor of his mouth that does not respond to conservative therapy. The patient has a history of smoking (one pack per day) and drinking two shots of gin a day for 30 years. Medically, the patient has rheumatoid arthritis and is being treated with multiple anti-inflammatory agents (i.e., aspirin, endomethacin, butazolidin).
Rating ______

Case #4—This 12-year-old patient presents with a gingival lesion (see Plate III, Fig. 74). A review of the patient's medical history reveals mumps at the age of nine, chicken pox at the age of six, and measles about the age of five. There is no other significant medical history.
Rating ______

Answers:

1)-3; 2)-1; 3)-3; 4)-0.

2. Malignant Potential

As the malignant potential of a lesion increases, so does the degree of surgical difficulty. The following factors must be considered before a surgical specimen is removed from a lesion with any malignant potential:

- ✓ You must be certain to do a thorough lymph node examination to locate and record any inflammatory or metastatic nodes.
- ✓ You must extend the surgical margin of the biopsy at least 0.5 cm beyond the clinical margin of the lesion due to the ability of tumors to extend beyond their apparent clinical margin.
- ✓ You may need to take multiple incisional biopsies in irregular lesions to ascertain areas of malignancy.
- ✓ You must realize that incisional biopsies are not always indicated for lesions over 1 cm when there is a high potential for malignancy. Such lesions are best treated by surgical excision and/or irradiation. These cases probably require the skills and experience of a trained specialist.

The rating scale for malignant potential has been divided into the following categories:

0—no malignant potential

1—low possibility of premalignancy in your differential diagnosis

2—premalignancy is a significant factor in your differential diagnosis

3—high degree of malignant potential

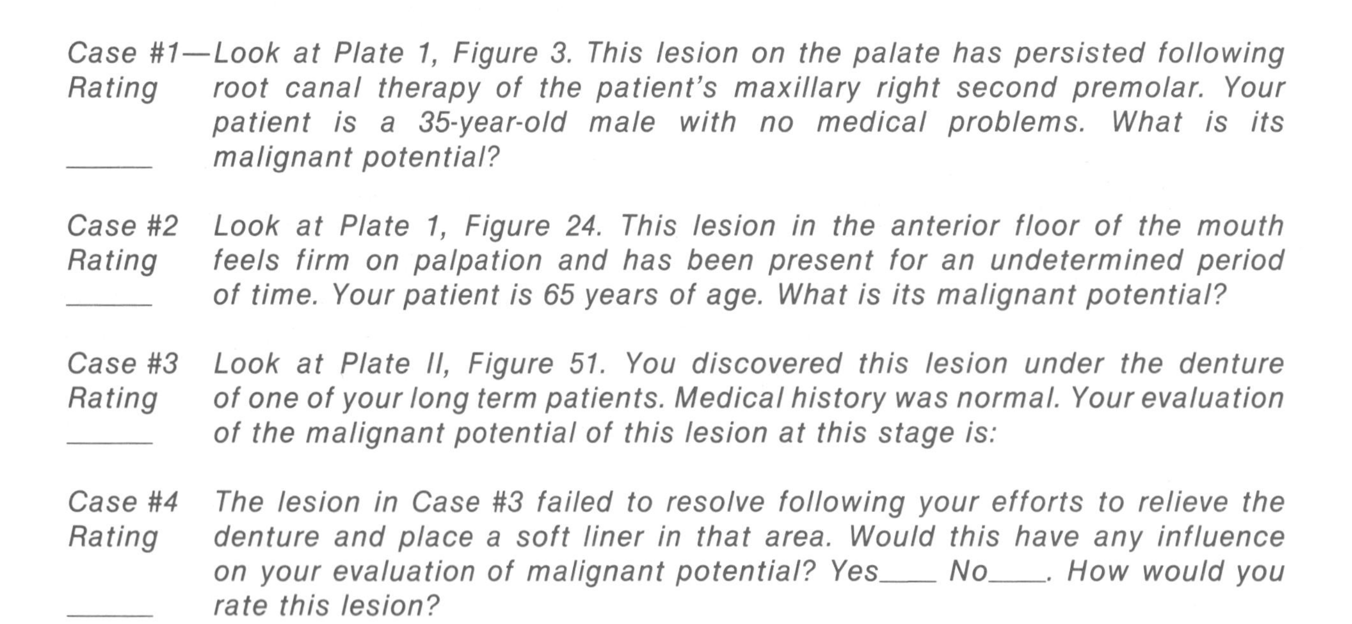

Case #1—Look at Plate 1, Figure 3. This lesion on the palate has persisted following
Rating root canal therapy of the patient's maxillary right second premolar. Your patient is a 35-year-old male with no medical problems. What is its
_____ malignant potential?

Case #2 Look at Plate 1, Figure 24. This lesion in the anterior floor of the mouth
Rating feels firm on palpation and has been present for an undetermined period
_____ of time. Your patient is 65 years of age. What is its malignant potential?

Case #3 Look at Plate II, Figure 51. You discovered this lesion under the denture
Rating of one of your long term patients. Medical history was normal. Your evaluation
_____ of the malignant potential of this lesion at this stage is:

Case #4 The lesion in Case #3 failed to resolve following your efforts to relieve the
Rating denture and place a soft liner in that area. Would this have any influence on your evaluation of malignant potential? Yes____ No____. How would you
_____ rate this lesion?

Answers:

1)-0; 2)-3; 3)-1; 4)-2.

3. Physical Properties of Tissue

Lesions have physical properties other than size which influence the degree of surgical difficulty. These properties can require you to modify your surgical technique and can influence not only what area of a lesion is sampled but whether you refer the patient to a specialist.

In Unit II you learned how to modify your surgical procedure according to the clinical appearance of the lesion. Here you will learn to assess the significance of eight major characteristics of lesions which contribute to the degree of difficulty. You should carefully evaluate each of the physical properties listed below for their influence on surgical procedure and on your decision whether to refer to a specialist.

A. Definition of margins (borders)

B. Surface characteristics

C. Depth of extension

D. Quality of tissue

E. Pigmentation

F. Vascularity

G. Soft tissue or bone

H. Growth rate

There is no implied order of importance to the above characteristics. Each characteristic contributes in a cumulative way such that the sum of the many factors could make the total procedure very difficult.

We will now examine each of the physical properties and develop criteria for rating their contribution. With the ability to consistently rate the eight properties, you can make an overall evaluation of the combined effects of all factors.

A. Definition of Margins (Borders)

How well a lesion is clinically delineated from the surrounding normal tissue influences the surgical difficulty. Clinically, it is more difficult to select an adequate surgical margin when the lesion has an indistinct border. **This requires that you extend the surgical margin beyond the usual 2 mm to ensure that you include a margin of normal tissue.** Examples include inflammatory and neoplastic processes which histologically extend beyond the apparent clinical margins. You may wish to refer back to Unit II, Site Selection, if this point is not clear.

The following criteria have been made in increasing order of surgical difficulty.

0 = well circumscribed margins

1 = circumscribed with focally indistinct margins

2 = indistinct margins

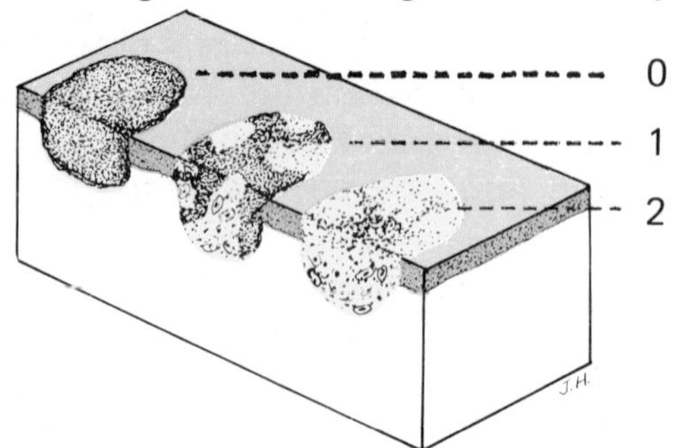

Figure III-2. Definition of Lesion Margins

B. Surface Characteristics

The surface characteristics will not influence your surgery if the lesion is small enough to be removed by excisional technique. **But with the incisional technique, the difficulty of selecting an adequate surgical site increases with rougher, more irregular, or more ulcerated surfaces.** These characteristics are also important in developing a differential diagnosis.

0 = surface contiguous with surrounding normal tissue

1 = moderately irregular surface (compared to surrounding normal tissue)

2 = severely rough and/or irregular or ulcerated surface

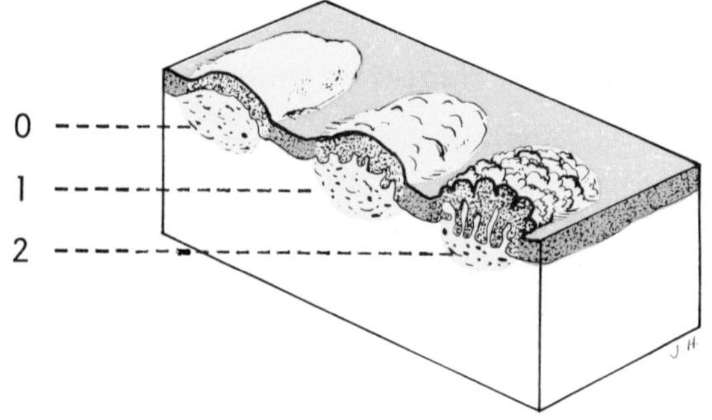

Figure III-3. Surface Characteristics

Remember, biopsies should include more than ulcerated area.

C. Depth of Extension

Lesions will have varying depths of extension. Superficial lesions will require no modification in surgical technique. But some lesions will extend deep into the subjacent structures (i.e., fat, skeletal muscle, bone). **These lesions require that you remove a deeper specimen, increasing the degree of difficulty.**

0 = superficial, involving epithelium and lamina propria

1 = extending into connective tissue

2 = extending into connective tissue and involving deeper structures, such as muscle, bone, fat and salivary glands.

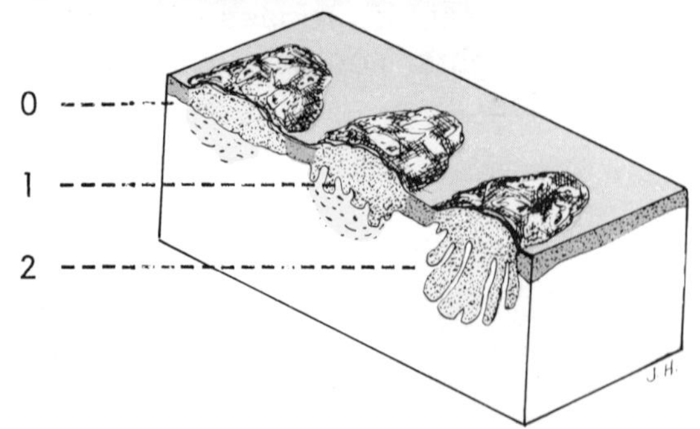

Figure III-4. Depth of Extension

D. Quality of Lesion

Some lesions are necrotic, friable, erosive, or bulbous-vesicular in nature. **These lesions require special attention as to surgical outline and handling technique.** In the rating scale below, we have divided the lesion into either normal tissue or necrotic, friable, **vesicular** components. In the diagram, "A" represents tissue of relatively normal consistency for both epithelial and connective tissue. "B" represents the "friable portion" area of necrosis, vesicle, or erosion. The ratio of B:A will tell you what percentage of the lesion has the "friable," or poor quality, component. The difficulty for obtaining a good specimen increases as the percentage of poor quality increases.

0 = tissue normal quality (0% B)

1 = less than 50% of the diameter of the lesion is of poor quality—B/A ⩽50%

2 = more than 50% of the diameter of the lesion is of poor quality—B/A ⩾50%

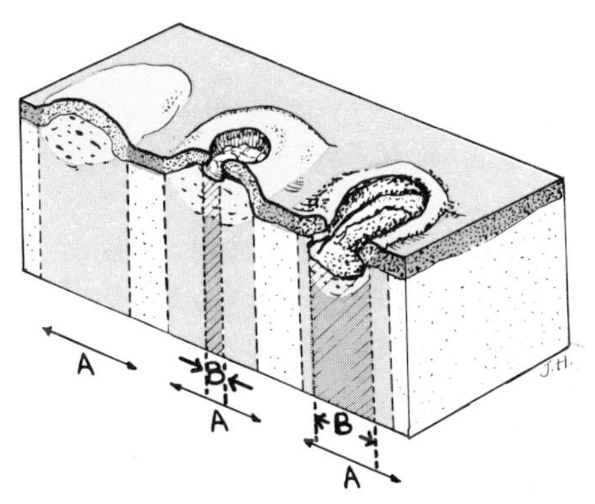

Figure III-5. Lesions of Poor Quality

E. Pigmentation

As you should recall from Unit II, **excisional biopsies of pigmented lesions may be performed, but incisions should not be made into the lesion.** Lesions which have an apparent extrinsic etiology, such as amalgam tattoo, require the removal of the usual margin of normal tissue. Those lesions that have an unknown etiology or those that show a rapid increase in size, require a wider margin. Thus, the degree of difficulty increases rapidly.

0 = non-pigmented

1 = pigmentation of long standing or definite extrinsic etiology (e.g., amalgam tattoo)

2 = pigmentation of unknown etiology or duration

3 = pigmentation of short history or sudden change in color or size

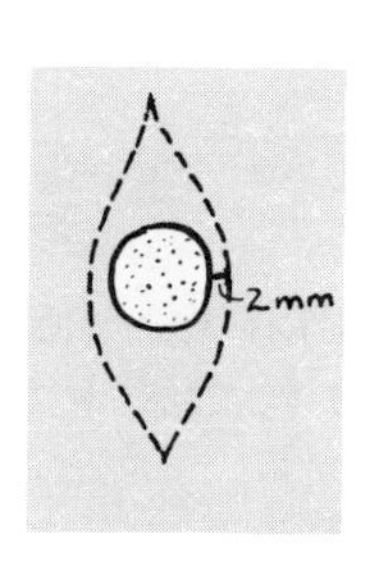

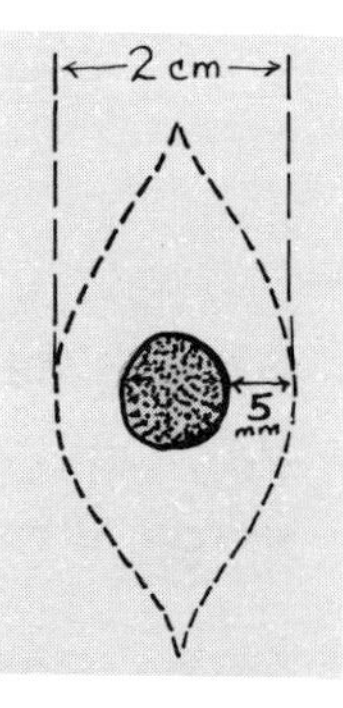

Figure III-6. Pigmented Lesions

The two lesions shown above are 10 mm (1.0 cm) in size. You must make the decision on whether to refer for biopsy. One is pigmented, the other is not. When biopsying pigmented lesions, you should extend your incision to 5 mm on either side. In doing this, you have increased your width to 20 mm for the pigmented lesion. This is a very large tissue sample and would be **considerably** more difficult than the 14 mm wide tissue sample required from the non-pigmented lesion.

F. Vascularity

As you remember from Unit II, **lesions which are entirely vascular in nature should not be sampled by the incisional technique.**

In general, the extension of the surgical margin must increase **as the degree of vascularity increases in both inflammatory and neoplastic lesions.** This increases the degree of surgical difficulty proportionally.

0 = no abnormal vascular component

1 = associated hyperemia

2 = abnormal vascular component within lesion (angiofibroma)

3 = lesion entirely vascular in nature (hemangiomas, vascular hamartomas)

G. Soft Tissue or Bone

As the amount of bony involvement increases so does the degree of difficulty.

0 = soft tissue

1 = soft tissue eroding bone

2 = soft tissue and bone involvement

3 = entirely bony (central) lesion

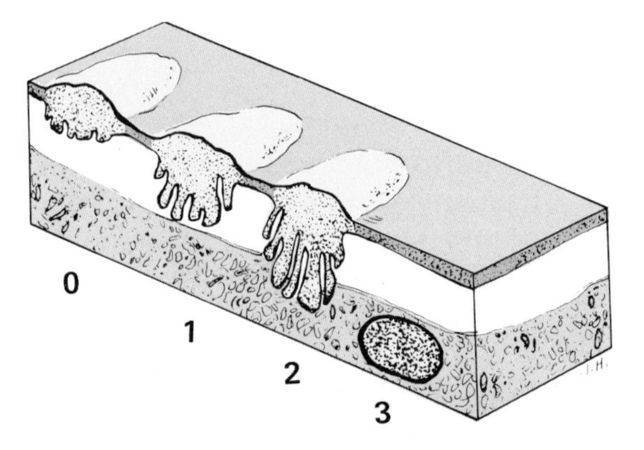

Figure III-7. The Degree of Difficulty Increases As More Bone Becomes Involved

H. Growth Rate

You will recall that **for more rapidly growing lesions you should extend your surgical margins further into apparently normal tissue.**

0 = no growth

1 = slow growth (months to years)

2 = moderate growth (weeks to months)

3 = rapid growth (days to weeks)

STUDY EXERCISES

Using the Evaluation Form and Summary Key Sheet, rate each of the lesions described as to their physical characteristics.

Case #1. *This lesion (see Plate I, Figure 9) has enlarged over the last year. The lesion does not appear to extend into the subjacent structures upon palpation.*

	0	1	2	3	Comments
A. Definition of Margins	☐	☐	☐		
B. Surface Characteristics	☐	☐	☐		
C. Depth of Extension	☐	☐	☐		
D. Quality of Tissue	☐	☐	☐		
E. Pigmentation	☐	☐	☐	☐	
F. Vascularity	☐	☐	☐	☐	
G. Soft Tissue or Bone	☐	☐	☐	☐	
H. Growth Rate	☐	☐	☐	☐	

Case #2. *This lesion (see Plate III, Figure 74) has been present at least six months. The lesion is superficial upon palpation.*

	0	1	2	3	Comments
A. Definition of Margins	☐	☐	☐		
B. Surface Characteristics	☐	☐	☐		
C. Depth of Extension	☐	☐	☐		
D. Quality of Tissue	☐	☐	☐		
E. Pigmentation	☐	☐	☐	☐	
F. Vascularity	☐	☐	☐	☐	
G. Soft Tissue or Bone	☐	☐	☐	☐	
H. Growth Rate	☐	☐	☐	☐	

Case #3. *These two lesions (see Plate II, Figure 29), have appeared and reached this size in two months, according to the patient. They appear slightly raised and firm to palpation.*

	0	1	2	3	Comments
A. Definition of Margins	☐	☐	☐		
B. Surface Characteristics	☐	☐	☐		
C. Depth of Extension	☐	☐	☐		
D. Quality of Tissue	☐	☐	☐		
E. Pigmentation	☐	☐	☐	☐	
F. Vascularity	☐	☐	☐	☐	
F. Soft Tissue or Bone	☐	☐	☐	☐	
G. Growth Rate	☐	☐	☐	☐	

Case #4. *This lesion (see Plate I, Figure 25), has been present for one year. The mesial raised area has appeared over a two week period and* ***bleeds*** *upon manipulation. The distal portion is slightly raised and* ***firm*** *to palpation. If you feel more than one specimen should be removed, rate each site separately.*

	0	1	2	3	Comments
A. Definition of Margins	☐	☐	☐		
B. Surface Characteristics	☐	☐	☐		
C. Depth of Extension	☐	☐	☐		
D. Quality of Tissue	☐	☐	☐		
E. Pigmentation	☐	☐	☐	☐	
F. Vascularity	☐	☐	☐	☐	
G. Soft Tissue or Bone	☐	☐	☐	☐	
H. Growth Rate	☐	☐	☐	☐	

STUDY EXERCISES—Answers

Case #1

	0	1	2	3
A. Definition of Margins	☐	☒	☐	
B. Surface Characteristics	☐	☒	☐	
C. Depth of Extension	☒	☐	☐	
D. Quality of Tissue	☒	☐	☐	
E. Pigmentation	☒	☐	☐	☐
F. Vascularity	☒	☐	☐	☐
G. Soft Tissue or Bone	☒	☐	☐	☐
H. Growth Rate	☐	☒	☐	☐

Comments
Considering the overall physical characteristics of this lesion, this lesion would not present any major difficulties for obtaining a good tissue specimen. However, you need to evaluate the other criteria for a true picture of the degree of difficulty.

Case #2

	0	1	2	3
A. Definition of Margins	☒	☐	☐	
B. Surface Characteristics	☐	☐	☒	
C. Depth of Extension	☒	☐	☐	
D. Quality of Tissue	☒	☐	☐	
E. Pigmentation	☒	☐	☐	☐
F. Vascularity	☒	☐	☐	☐
G. Soft Tissue or Bone	☒	☐	☐	☐
H. Growth Rate	☐	☒	☐	☐

Comments
The only physical property of this lesion that might be of concern is the surface character.

Case #3

	0	1	2	3
A. Definition of Margins	☐	☒	☐	
B. Surface Characteristics	☒	☐	☐	
C. Depth of Extension	☒	☐	☐	
D. Quality of Tissue	☒	☐	☐	
E. Pigmentation	☐	☐	☐	☒
F. Vascularity	☒	☐	☐	☐
G. Soft Tissue or Bone	☒	☐	☐	☐
H. Growth Rate	☐	☐	☒	☐

Comments
Both pigmentation and growth rate show up to be significant complicating factors.

Case #4

	0	1	2	3
A. Definition of Margins	☒	☐	☐	
B. Surface Characteristics	☐	☐	☒	
C. Depth of Extension	☐	☒	☐	
D. Quality of Tissue	☐	☒	☒	
E. Pigmentation	☒	☐	☐	☐
F. Vascularity	☐	☐	☒	☐
G. Soft Tissue or Bone	☒	☐	☐	☐
H. Growth Rate	☒	☐	☐	☒

Comments
This lesion shows two areas that differ in physical properties. The mesial area (M) shows a higher malignant potential as well as tissue of a poorer overall quality. The distal area (D) shows to be of better quality.

I. Overall Effects of Physical Properties of Lesions on the Degree of Difficulty for Biopsy Procedures.

A rating system for the physical properties of oral lesions provides useful information as to the **overall effect** of the lesion on the surgical technique required for collection of an adequate tissue specimen. The higher the "score" the more the physical properties of the lesion affect the overall surgical difficulty. The effects this can have on the surgical procedure include:

- Increasing the overall size of the wound area.
- Increasing the depth of the wound.

As the size of the wound increases in both surface area and depth, the higher the surgeon's training level required to effectively manage the procedure.

As a guideline for determining the overall effect of the physical properties, the following categories have been arbitrarily defined:

0 = all ratings in the "0" category

1 = all ratings in the "0" or "1" category

2 = all ratings in the "0" or "1" or "2" category (if more than two "2"s, this should be a "3").

3 = any "3"s or more than two "2"s

STUDY EXERCISES

For each of the following cases, evaluate the overall effect of physical properties on the degree of surgical difficulty. Also, state the major factors that influence this overall evaluation.

#1

Pre-Surgical Evaluation:	**0**	**1**	**2**	**3**
1. Patient's general health	☒	☐	☐	☐
2. Malignant potential	☒	☐	☐	☐
3. Physical properties				
A. Definition of margins	☐	☒	☐	
B. Surface characteristics	☐	☒	☐	
C. Depth of extension	☒	☐	☐	
D. Quality of tissue	☒	☐	☐	
E. Pigmentation	☒	☐	☐	☐
F. Vascularity	☒	☐	☐	☐
G. Soft tissue or bone	☒	☐	☐	☐
H. Growth rate	☐	☒	☐	☐
I. Overall effect of physical properties	☐	☐	☐	☐

Major Factors: ______________________

____

____

#2

Pre-Surgical Evaluation:	**0**	**1**	**2**	**3**
1. Patient's general health	☒	☐	☐	☐
2. Malignant potential	☒	☐	☐	☐
3. Physical properties				
A. Definition of margins	☒	☐	☐	
B. Surface characteristics	☐	☐	☒	
C. Depth of extension	☒	☐	☐	
D. Quality of tissue	☒	☐	☐	
E. Pigmentation	☒	☐	☐	☐
F. Vascularity	☒	☐	☐	☐
G. Soft tissue or bone	☒	☐	☐	☐
H. Growth rate	☐	☒	☐	☐
I. Overall effect of physical properties	☐	☐	☐	☐

Major Factors: ______________________

____

____

STUDY EXERCISES—continued

#3

Pre-Surgical Evaluation:	**0**	**1**	**2**	**3**
1. Patient's general health	☒	☐	☐	☐
2. Malignant potential	☒	☐	☐	☐
3. Physical properties				
A. Definition of margins	☐	☒	☐	
B. Surface characteristics	☒	☐	☐	
C. Depth of extension	☒	☐	☐	
D. Quality of tissue	☒	☐	☐	
E. Pigmentation	☐	☐	☐	☒
F. Vascularity	☒	☐	☐	☐
G. Soft tissue or bone	☒	☐	☐	☐
H. Growth rate	☐	☐	☒	☐
I. Overall effect of physical properties	☐	☐	☐	☐

Major Factors: ______________________________

____

____

#4

Pre-Surgical Evaluation:	**0**	**1**	**2**	**3**
1. Patient's general health	☒	☐	☐	☐
2. Malignant potential	☒	☐	☐	☐
3. Physical properties				
A. Definition of margins	☒	☐	☐	
B. Surface characteristics	☐	☐	☒	
C. Depth of extension	☐	☒	☐	
D. Quality of tissue	☐	☒	☒	
E. Pigmentation	☒	☐	☐	☐
F. Vascularity	☐	☐	☒	☐
G. Soft tissue or bone	☒	☐	☐	☐
H. Growth rate	☒	☐	☐	☒
I. Overall effect of physical properties	☐	☐	☐	☐

Major Factors: ______________________________

____

____

STUDY EXERCISES—Answers

1. The overall effect of physical properties of this lesion would be a "1" and would not present any major problems in removing an adequate specimen.

2. Although this lesion has severely irregular surface characteristics ("2"), other characteristics present no problems. Thus, the overall rating is a "2" but it would be a weak "2".

3. In this case, the presence of dark pigmentation ("3") in addition to a moderate growth rate ("2") would place the overall effects in the "3" category. This should be referred to an oral surgeon or other specialist.

4. In this case, surface characteristics ("2"), quality of tissue ("2"), vascularity ("2"), and rapid growth ("3"), all combine to make this a difficult ("3") situation. Referral is definitely indicated here.

4. Size of the Lesion

We stated in Unit II that lesions smaller than 1 cm are usually surgically excised (excisional technique). We also stated that lesions larger than 1 cm are most often sampled by the incisional technique. The difficulty of tissue removal increases with an increase in size of the lesion. Therefore, the following scale has been developed to provide you with a method for evaluating the effect of increased size on surgical difficulty.

0 = less than 0.5 cm (excisional biopsy technique)

1 = .5 - 1.0 cm (excisional biopsy technique)

2 = 1.0 cm + requiring only one incisional biopsy and lesions well localized

3 = 1.0 cm + requiring multiple incisional biopsies (lesion not well localized and irregular in texture and outline)

STUDY EXERCISE

For each of the cases below, rate the difficulty according to lesion size.

Picture	Size	0	1	2	3
Case 1 Plate I, Fig. 3	*4 mm*	☐	☐	☐	☐
Case 2 Plate I, Fig. 24	*2 x 2 cm*	☐	☐	☐	☐
Case 3 Plate I, Fig. 25	*10 x 15 cm*	☐	☐	☐	☐
Case 4 Plate I, Fig. 26	*9.0 x 13 mm (not torus)*	☐	☐	☐	☐
Case 5 Plate I, Fig. 5	*0.8 mm*	☐	☐	☐	☐

STUDY EXERCISE—Answers

Case 1 = 0; Case 2 = 3; Case 3 = 3; Case 4 = 2; Case 5 = 1

5. Degree of Surgical Access

The usual definition of access implies an ability to see and reach an area for surgery. However, you must also include anatomic structures adjacent to the surgical area and your ability to stabilize the surgical site during the specific biopsy technique.

For example, if we compare the process of removing a small papilloma from the buccal attached gingivae adjacent to a maxillary first premolar with the removal of a similar lesion located on the posterior floor of the mouth, the latter lesion will be much more difficult to remove because it is:

- Harder to see
- Harder to reach
- Harder to stabilize during the surgery
- Associated with complex underlying anatomy

The following rating system will help you to identify potential difficulties with surgical access. The involved factors, already alluded to, include:

- **Ability to see the lesion.**
- **Ability to reach the lesion.**
- **Ability to stabilize the lesion.**
- **Ability to avoid underlying anatomy.**

We will examine each of the above factors and specify a rating system to show the relationships between factors and how they can compound to create a greater level of complexity.

A. Ability to See the Lesion

The more difficult it is to see the lesion, the more trouble you will have obtaining an adequate tissue sample. The rating scale has been divided into the following categories:

0 = direct unobstructed vision.

1 = requires minor manipulation of tissue or patient position.

2 = indirect vision with a mirror **or** tongue or cheek retraction.

3 = indirect vision with mirror required **as well as** retraction of tongue or cheek.

STUDY EXERCISES

For each of the lesions below, rate your ABILITY TO SEE THE LESION.

Case	*0*	*1*	*2*	*3*	*Comments*
1. Plate I, Fig. 13	☐	☐	☐	☐	______
2. Plate I, Fig. 25	☐	☐	☐	☐	______
3. Plate I, Fig. 3	☐	☐	☐	☐	______
4. Plate III, Fig. 70	☐	☐	☐	☐	______

STUDY EXERCISES—Answers

1)-3; 2)-2; 3)-0; 4)-1.

B. Ability to Reach the Lesion

Often you can see lesions in locations that are hard to reach with your surgical instruments. This can greatly increase the difficulty you will have in obtaining an acceptable tissue specimen.

The rating scale has been divided into the following categories:

0—direct unobstructed instrument approach possible.

1—requires minor manipulation of tissue or patient position in order to reach lesion with a direct approach.

2—minor tongue or cheek retraction **or** slight modifications in surgical technique required to reach the lesion.

3—major tissue or tongue retraction necessary **as well as** modifications in normal instrument utilization.

STUDY EXERCISES

For each of the cases below, rate your ability to reach the lesion with the standard biopsy instruments.

Case	*0*	*1*	*2*	*3*	*Comments*
1. Plate II, Fig. 34	☐	☐	☐	☐	________
2. Plate I, Fig. 9	☐	☐	☐	☐	________
3. Plate I, Fig. 13	☐	☐	☐	☐	________
4. Plate III, Fig. 72	☐	☐	☐	☐	________

STUDY EXERCISES—Answers

1)—0; 2)—3; 3)—3; 4)—2.

C. Ability to Stabilize the Lesion

It is generally easier to secure an acceptable tissue specimen when you have an immobile surgical site. It is easier to sample a soft lesion overlying bone than a lesion with soft movable tissue underlying it. It is generally easier to secure a tissue specimen from attached gingivae than from the soft palate, cheek, tongue, or floor of the mouth.

The rating scale has been divided into the following categories:

0 = tissue not mobile—attached gingiva or hard palate.

1 = movable tissue with underlying bone—alveolar mucosa.

2 = soft tissue that can be easily immobilized by the operator—lips, buccal mucosa (cheek), anterior one-third of the tongue.

3 = very difficult to stabilize tissue, requires modification in basic technique. Soft palate floor of mouth, ventral surface of tongue, anterior pillars.

STUDY EXERCISES

For each of the cases below, rate the ability to stabilize the tissue for surgery.

Case	*0*	*1*	*2*	*3*	*Comments*
1. Plate 1, Fig. 3	☐	☐	☐	☐	__________
2. Plate II, Fig. 51	☐	☐	☐	☐	__________
3. Plate III, Fig. 77	☐	☐	☐	☐	__________
4. Plate I, Fig. 10	☐	☐	☐	☐	__________

STUDY EXERCISES—Answers

1)—0; 2)—1; 3)—2; 4)—3.

D. Underlying Anatomy

During the surgical removal of diseased tissue for pathological examination, you also have to consider adjacent or underlying anatomic structures. These structures may include blood vessels, nerves, muscle, and salivary glands and ducts. **Therefore, removal of similar lesions from different anatomic locations will have different degrees of difficulty due to the varying potential for damage to underlying structures.**

The rating scale has been divided into the following categories:

0 = no significant underlying structures (attached gingiva on mandible anterior to second molar and buccal of maxillary arch)

1 = underlying anatomic structures that would not preclude surgery in that area (buccal mucosa, lower lip, dorsal surface of tongue)

2 = significant anatomic structures are adjacent to the area of surgery but can be avoided by awareness of structures and modification of surgical technique (around mental nerve, greater palatine foramen incisive canal, lesion in bone close to inferior alveolar nerve)

3 = multiple significant adjacent anatomic structures within the surgical bed which could cause permanent injury or a surgical emergency (i.e., incising the facial artery), or the lesion involves major anatomic structures (floor of the mouth contains nerves, blood vessels, salivary ducts, and muscle attachments)

STUDY EXERCISES

Rate the following cases as to significant underlying anatomy. Name the structures that may be injured during the surgical procedure. You may desire to use your gross anatomy or oral anatomy reference books.

Case	*0*	*1*	*2*	*3*	*Underlying Structures Involved*
1. Plate 1, Fig. 2	☐	☐	☐	☐	__________
2. Plate 1, Fig. 24	☐	☐	☐	☐	__________
3. Plate I, Fig. 25	☐	☐	☐	☐	__________
4. Plate I, Fig. 26	☐	☐	☐	☐	__________
5. Plate III, Fig. 73	☐	☐	☐	☐	__________

STUDY EXERCISES—*Answers*

Rating Structures

1. *0—None*
2. *2*
3. *3—Lingual nerve, long buccal nerve*
4. *3—Greater palatine, NAV cannot be avoided in removing this lesion.*
5. *2—Mental nerve*

STUDY EXERCISES

Now rate the following lesions for ease of surgical access, using the key provided at the end of the chapter. Comment on anticipated problems.

Case #1 See Plate I, Fig. 3

Surgical Access	*Rating Scale* 0	1	2	3	*Comments*
A. Ability to See	☐	☐	☐	☐	________
B. Ability to Reach	☐	☐	☐	☐	________
C. Ability to Stabilize	☐	☐	☐	☐	________
D. Underlying Anatomy	☐	☐	☐	☐	________

Case #2 See Plate I, Fig. 9

Surgical Access	0	1	2	3	*Comments*
A. Ability to See	☐	☐	☐	☐	________
B. Ability to Reach	☐	☐	☐	☐	________
C. Ability to Stabilize	☐	☐	☐	☐	________
D. Underlying Anatomy	☐	☐	☐	☐	________

Case #3 See Plate I, Fig. 13

Surgical Access	0	1	2	3	*Comments*
A. Ability to See	☐	☐	☐	☐	________
B. Ability to Reach	☐	☐	☐	☐	________
C. Ability to Stabilize	☐	☐	☐	☐	________
D. Underlying Anatomy	☐	☐	☐	☐	________

STUDY EXERCISES—*Answers*

1. *A-0; B-0; C-0; D-0.*
   This should be an easy surgery. No categories reveal complicating factors.
2. *A-2; B-2; C-3; D-3.*
   Surgical access difficult. Sight and reach present some problems, but stabilization and underlying anatomy create significant difficulties.
3. *A-3; B-3; C-3; D-3.*
   All factors show this to be a very difficult surgery. Most dentists would take one look and refer this lesion.

6. Overall Degree of Difficulty

You now have considerable experience evaluating the many factors that contribute to overall surgical difficulty for removing a tissue specimen for histopathological examination. How can this information be used in deciding whether to do the surgery yourself or refer to someone with more experience? Two things need to be kept in mind:

- The absolute numerical evaluation of each factor and overall difficulty.
- The type of surgical procedures you routinely perform in your own office.

■ Numerical Evaluation

We have adjusted the numerical values for each factor so that the range of categories would lie within the capabilities of most general practitioners. Any factor with a "0" rating would generally present little problem to a general practitioner. However, any factor evaluated as "3" could complicate the surgery enough to be beyond the ability of most general practitioners.

If an evaluation reveals multiple factors in the "3" category, you are dealing with a very difficult situation.

In the middle range ("1"s and "2"s), you need to look at the aggregate or synergistic effect of multiple factors. It is possible that a surgery evaluated as all "2"s could be **more** difficult than a similar surgery in which a "3" factor was accompanied by "0"s and "1"s.

Example: If you have a very small (rating "0" for size) hemangioma, rating "3" for vascularity and rating "0"s for all four access factors, you may be dealing with a surgical situation within your capabilities. In this case you would be inclined to rate the overall difficulty as a "2" rather than the "3" indicated by the vascularity. Be careful **NOT** to over-rationalize this interpretation.

General Guideline for Numerical Evaluation

- **Generally speaking, the overall evaluation is the same as the HIGHEST rated single factor.**
- **A "3" in overall difficulty usually implies referral is indicated.**
- **If you find multiple factors in the "2" column, INCREASE the overall rating to "3".**

Your Office Routine

Your final criteria for referral should relate to the kinds of surgery you perform on a routine basis in your office.

If you usually do no surgery, even a lesion evaluated to be all "0" could be a traumatic experience for both you and your patient.

If you routinely reflect flaps for extraction of teeth or for pre-prosthetic surgery, you could feel relatively secure performing surgery for cases with over-all ratings of "0," "1," and "2," again depending upon the specific case.

If you routinely treat large lesions in hard-to-reach areas and have had special training in dissecting the floor of the mouth, in dealing with severe medical problems, and in surgical management of malignancies, then, of course, you probably have the skills and experience to manage cases with one or more "3" evaluations.

In summary, your decision to refer should be based upon accurate evaluation of the case, matched to your level of experience and the physical set-up in your office.

STUDY EXERCISES

Evaluate the overall degree of difficulty for each of the following cases. Explain the reasons for your answers.

Pre-Surgical Evaluation:

Evaluate the overall degree of difficulty for each of the cases.

Case #1
See Plate I, Fig. 9.

	0	1	2	3
1. Patient's general health	☐	☒	☐	☐
2. Malignant potential	☐	☐	☒	☐
3. Physical properties				
A. Definition of margins	☐	☒	☐	
B. Surface characteristics	☐	☒	☐	
C. Depth of extension	☒	☐	☐	
D. Quality of tissue	☒	☐	☐	
E. Pigmentation	☒	☐	☐	☐
F. Vascularity	☒	☐	☐	☐
G. Soft tissue or bone	☒	☐	☐	☐
H. Growth rate	☐	☐	☒	☐
I. Overall effect of physical properties	☐	☐	☒	☐
4. Size of lesion	☐	☐	☐	☒
5. Degree of surgical access				
A. Ability to see	☐	☐	☒	☐
B. Ability to reach	☐	☐	☐	☒
C. Ability to stabilize	☐	☐	☐	☒
D. Underlying anatomy	☐	☐	☐	☒
★ **6. Overall difficulty**	☐	☐	☐	☐

Explain your choice.

STUDY EXERCISES

Pre-Surgical Evaluation:

Case #2
See Plate III,
Fig. 74.

Explain your choice.

	0	1	2	3
1. Patient's general health	☒	☐	☐	☐
2. Malignant potential	☒	☐	☐	☐
3. Physical properties				
A. Definition of margins	☒	☐	☐	
B. Surface characteristics	☐	☒	☐	
C. Depth of extension	☒	☐	☐	
D. Quality of tissue	☒	☐	☐	
E. Pigmentation	☒	☐	☐	☐
F. Vascularity	☒	☐	☐	☐
G. Soft tissue or bone	☒	☐	☐	☐
H. Growth rate	☐	☒	☐	☐
I. Overall effect of physical properties	☐	☐	☐	☐
4. Size of lesion	☐	☒	☐	☐
5. Degree of surgical access				
A. Ability to see	☐	☒	☐	☐
B. Ability to reach	☐	☒	☐	☐
C. Ability to stabilize	☐	☐	☐	☐
D. Underlying anatomy	☐	☐	☐	☐
★ **6. Overall difficulty**	☐	☐	☐	☐

Pre-Surgical Evaluation:

Case #3
See Plate II,
Fig. 19.

Explain your choice.

	0	1	2	3
1. Patient's general health	☒	☐	☐	☐
2. Malignant potential	☐	☐	☒	☐
3. Physical properties				
A. Definition of margins	☐	☒	☐	
B. Surface characteristics	☒	☐	☐	
C. Depth of extension	☒	☐	☐	
D. Quality of tissue	☒	☐	☐	
E. Pigmentation	☐	☐	☐	☒
F. Vascularity	☒	☐	☐	☐
G. Soft tissue or bone	☒	☐	☐	☐
H. Growth rate	☐	☐	☒	☐
I. Overall effect of physical properties	☐	☐	☐	☒
4. Size of lesion	☐	☒	☐	☐
5. Degree of surgical access				
A. Ability to see	☐	☐	☒	☐
B. Ability to reach	☐	☐	☒	☐
C. Ability to stabilize	☒	☐	☐	☐
D. Underlying anatomy	☐	☐	☒	☐
★ **6. Overall difficulty**	☐	☐	☐	☐

STUDY EXERCISES—Answers

1. *Overall difficulty—"3". Despite the fact that the overall effect of physical properties is a "1," the remaining factors, malignant potential, size, and degree of surgical access combine to make this a very difficult problem.*
2. *Overall difficulty—"1". Because the majority of factors were evaluated at "1" or below, with the exception of physical properties, an overall difficulty of "1" was assigned.*
3. *Overall difficulty—"3". Because of a "3" rating for physical properties and ratings of "2" in malignant potential and degree of surgical access, the overall difficulty rating is a "3".*

Now retake pre-test and proceed to Unit IV

UNIT IV

WHAT TO DO WITH YOUR PATHOLOGIST'S REPORT

PRE-TEST—UNIT IV

- *Answer the following questions.*
- *Compare your answers with those on page 76.*
- *If all your responses were correct, you have finished this book.*
- *If only some of your responses were correct, you can profit by studying this unit.*

Questions:

1. *What should be your course of action if the pathology report does not agree with your clinical evaluation of the lesion you have just biopsied?* ______________________
____
____

2. *If you have a choice in referring your specimens to a general pathologist or an oral pathologist, whom would you choose?* ______________________
Why? ____
____

3. *Check which of the following terms are commonly used in the description of malignant conditions:*

______ a. *Acanthosis*
______ b. *Carcinoma*
______ c. *Adenocarcinoma*
______ d. *Dyskeratosis*
______ e. *Parakeratosis*
______ f. *Orderly*
______ g. *Invasive carcinoma*
______ h. *Hyperkeratosis*
______ i. *Inflammatory*
______ j. *Undifferentiated*

4. *What should be your course of treatment for lesions described as neoplastic and malignant?* ______________________
____

5. *What should be your course of action for lesions described as non-neoplastic-hyperkeratotic?* ______________________
____

6. *What should be your course of action for lesions described as being non-neoplastic-inflammatory?* ____________________

____

7. *What should be your course of action for lesions described as neoplastic-pre-malignant?* ____________________

____

8. *Although it is never pleasant to inform your patient of a malignant diagnosis, what specific things can you do to decrease the shock of the information?*

   a. ____________________
   b. ____________________
   c. ____________________
   d. ____________________

PRE-TEST—Unit IV, Answers

1. *If your clinical diagnosis or suspicion is that a lesion could be malignant, but your pathologist says the specimen examined did not show malignancy, you should submit another specimen from a different area of the lesion. (This usually applies to incisional specimens).*
2. *Oral pathologist. An oral pathologist has special training in oral conditions.*
3. *Malignant terms are: b, c, d, g, j.*
4. *Refer to tumor board or oral surgeon immediately.*
5. *This lesion should be removed by you or your oral surgeon.*
6. *You should first remove the etiology and observe for 7-14 days. If it does not improve, further referral may be needed.*
7. *You should refer this lesion to an oral surgeon for total removal. Generally, these lesions require wider surgical margins.*
8. *a. Discuss this with your patient's physician.*
   b. Let the tumor board or oral surgeon inform your patient.
   c. Emphasize the positive aspects of care and therapy.
   d. Tell only as much as the patient wants to know.

CONTENT FOR UNIT IV

WHAT TO DO WITH YOUR PATHOLOGIST'S REPORT

WHAT CAN I DO NOW?

Usually you will receive a written report from your pathologist within seven days. Once you receive the report, further action is up to you. At this time you must make the decision to:

- **Institute no further treatment, but follow the condition.**

- **Remove the remaining portion of the lesion (as in the case of incisional technique).**

- **Refer your patient to a specialist for further action involving:**
  Local surgery
  Radiation therapy
  Chemotherapy

As the general dentist, your primary role now is to interpret your pathologist's report and select the appropriate course of action. In this unit, we will provide you with criteria to help choose the appropriate course of action.

GENERAL CONSIDERATIONS

You may have a clinical diagnosis that occasionally is not in agreement with the pathologist's report. You may "feel" a lesion is malignant whereas the pathology report does not substantiate this clinical impression.

General Rules

- **If your pathologist's report agrees with your clinical diagnosis, proceed with the various treatment options.**

- **If the pathology report does not agree with your clinical diagnosis, submit another specimen.**

Remember, your pathologist can only interpret the lesion based on the clinical description and specimen you submit. His diagnosis can only be as accurate as the information he has available. **He is ADVISORY to your final diagnosis.**

Interpreting a biopsy report to determine whether a neoplastic or non-neoplastic lesion is benign, pre-malignant, or malignant can sometimes be difficult.

A GENERAL PATHOLOGIST who is very capable in his field sometimes neglects to distinguish between pre-malignant and benign oral entities. He may also fail to diagnose common non-neoplastic oral lesions (e.g., pyogenic granuloma, lichen planus, and others). He may also use the term leukoplakia vaguely, which makes it difficult for the referring dentist to determine the pre-malignant or benign character of the lesion. When even a shadow of a doubt arises in the mind of the referring dentist, a good suggestion is to call your pathologist and clarify terminology.

SUGGESTION: Whenever possible, submit samples of oral tissue to an **ORAL PATHOLOGIST.** The oral pathologist will usually give you an interpretation of whether the lesion:

- Is neoplastic or non-neoplastic.
- Is benign, pre-malignant, or malignant.

STUDY EXERCISES

1. *You have just received a pathology report from your local oral pathologist. The report states the tissue you submitted two days ago showed findings consistent with benign hyperkeratosis. However, when you submitted the specimen, you had a high suspicion of either a pre-malignant or malignant condition. The lesion was similar to that shown on Plate 1, Figure 9. You removed an incisional specimen from the ventral surface of the tongue. Describe what you should do now.* ________________

   ____

   Why? ________________________________

2. *Would your course of action be the same if your clinical impression was benign hyperkeratosis, but the pathology report indicated squamous cell carcinoma?*

   ____

   What would you do? ________________________________

   ____

3. *Why is it recommended that you send your specimens to a trained oral pathologist rather than a general pathologist?* ________________________________

   ____

TERMINOLOGY

Occasionally the terminology of a pathology report can be difficult to interpret. The following are the usual descriptive terms used in neoplastic and non-neoplastic diseases.

Neoplastic Lesions

Malignant Neoplasms

Microscopic Description

abnormal mitotic figures
hyperchromatism
premature keratinization
pleomorphism
loss of polarity
reversed nuclear/cytoplasmic ratio
invasive
disorderly
infiltrating
dyskeratotic
undifferentiated
anaplastic
streaming
dysplastic

Diagnosis

carcinoma
adenocarcinoma
______ sarcoma, such as:
angio-(vascular) rhabdo—(skeletal muscle)
lymphangio (lymphatic) leio—(smooth muscle)
neuro—(nerve)
lipo—(fat)
osteo—(bone)
chondro—(cartilage)
carcinoma-in-situ
invasive carcinoma
lymphoma
(lymphosarcoma)

Pre-malignant Neoplasms

Terms used to describe pre-malignant lesions are the same as those used to describe malignant lesions. In addition, the following terms may be used.

epithelial
atypia (mild, moderate, severe)
dysplasia
reactive

Benign Neoplasms

Microscopic Description

encapsulated
orderly
parakeratosis
pseudoepitheliomatous hyperplasia
focal keratosis
regular
hyperkeratosis
acanthosis reactive

Diagnosis

______ adenoma
papilloma
angioma
neurofibroma
lipoma
leiomyoma
myxoma
fibroma
lymphangeoma
schwannoma
rhabdomyoma
osteoma
chondroma

NOTE: Benign terms can be used in the description of a malignant lesion, but malignant terms are rarely if ever used in the description of a benign lesion.

Non-neoplastic Lesions

Terminology Used in Microscopic Descriptions

The terminology used in the microscopic description of all three categories of non-neoplastic lesions is similar and would contain such terms as those listed below.

acanthosis
hyperkeratotis
______ hyperplasia
granulation tissue
acute/chronic inflammation
  (including specific inflammatory cell types)
ulceration
fibrosis
scar formation
edema
extravisated red blood cells
______ metaplasia
atrophy
hypertrophy
necrosis
______ cyst (cystic)

Diagnostic Terms for Non-neoplastic Lesions

Similar terminology is used for "reactive" and "inflammatory" lesions in that both types are pathologic manifestations of the basic inflammatory response.

benign keratosis (hyperkeratosis)
denture irritation hyperplasia
papillary palatal hyperplasia
irritation fibroma
pyogenic granuloma
peripheral giant cell granuloma
chronic sclerosing osteomyelitis (condensing osteitis)

Terms used in the diagnosis of **systemic** problems that cause changes in oral tissue:

lichen planus
lupus erythematosus
dilantin hyperplasia
puberty gingivitis
pregnancy gingivitis (and tumor)
consistent with ______
  vitamin C deficiency
  diabetes mellitus
plemphigus vulgaris
benign mucous membrane pemphigoid
stomatitis medimentosa
erythema multiforme
amyloidosis

NOTE: Some terms commonly used for inflammatory or reactive processes may be confused with terms used for benign neoplasms. For example: irritation fibroma (fibroma durum), "hemangioma" in granulation tissue type, or "pregnancy tumor." Of course, if you are unfamiliar with the meaning of your pathologist's particular diagnosis, you should contact him and/or refer to your standard oral pathology reference texts.

OUTLINE FOR PATIENT MANAGEMENT BASED ON PATHOLOGIST'S REPORT

Introduction

After reading the pathologist's report, you must make those decisons that will result in the best possible management of your patient's problem. Should you have any problems in deciding on appropriate action, DO NOT HESITATE to call your pathologist or other specialists for assistance. If you are unclear about the terminology your pathologist uses, call him. If you are unclear about a surgical procedure that is necessary, call (or refer your patient to) an oral surgeon.

On page 82, we have presented a decision tree to assist you in selecting an appropriate course of action. The diagram and discussion are intended as a general guide. Specific cases may involve problems not discussed in this unit that would modify the procedures and process we describe. For cases outside the scope of this book, additional consultation or referral should be sought.

Philosophy Behind This Management System

Before employing any of the various treatment methods, you need to know the nature of the disease process and the extent of the problem.

Neoplastic lesions are usually managed differently than non-neoplastic lesions. We have presented a method for you to make this distinction in Criteria 1.

Benign, malignant and pre-malignant neoplastic lesions can be treated in different ways. Malignant and pre-malignant conditions should be referred to specialists AS SOON AS POSSIBLE. You may be able to remove benign neoplasms or you may wish to refer them to your oral surgeon, depending on the patient, size of lesion, location, and your surgical abilities.

Non-neoplastic lesions, be they reactive, inflammatory, or systemic in nature, also have various treatment options. You should be able to manage some of these. Others may require the assistance of other health care personnel, including oral surgeons, physicians, etc.

In utilizing this flow system, your first decision is to determine whether the lesion is neoplastic or non-neoplastic. This can usually be done by analysis of specific terminology used in the pathology report. (See terminology section of this unit.) If you cannot make this distinction, you should call your pathologist.

- **Neoplastic Lesions**

  If the lesion is neoplastic, the determination of benign, malignant, or pre-malignant should be in the report. If not, call your pathologist for clarification.

  - ☐ **Benign**

    If the lesion is benign, then the total lesion should be removed. If the surgery is within your ability, you can remove it. If you feel additional skills are required, refer your patient to an oral surgeon.

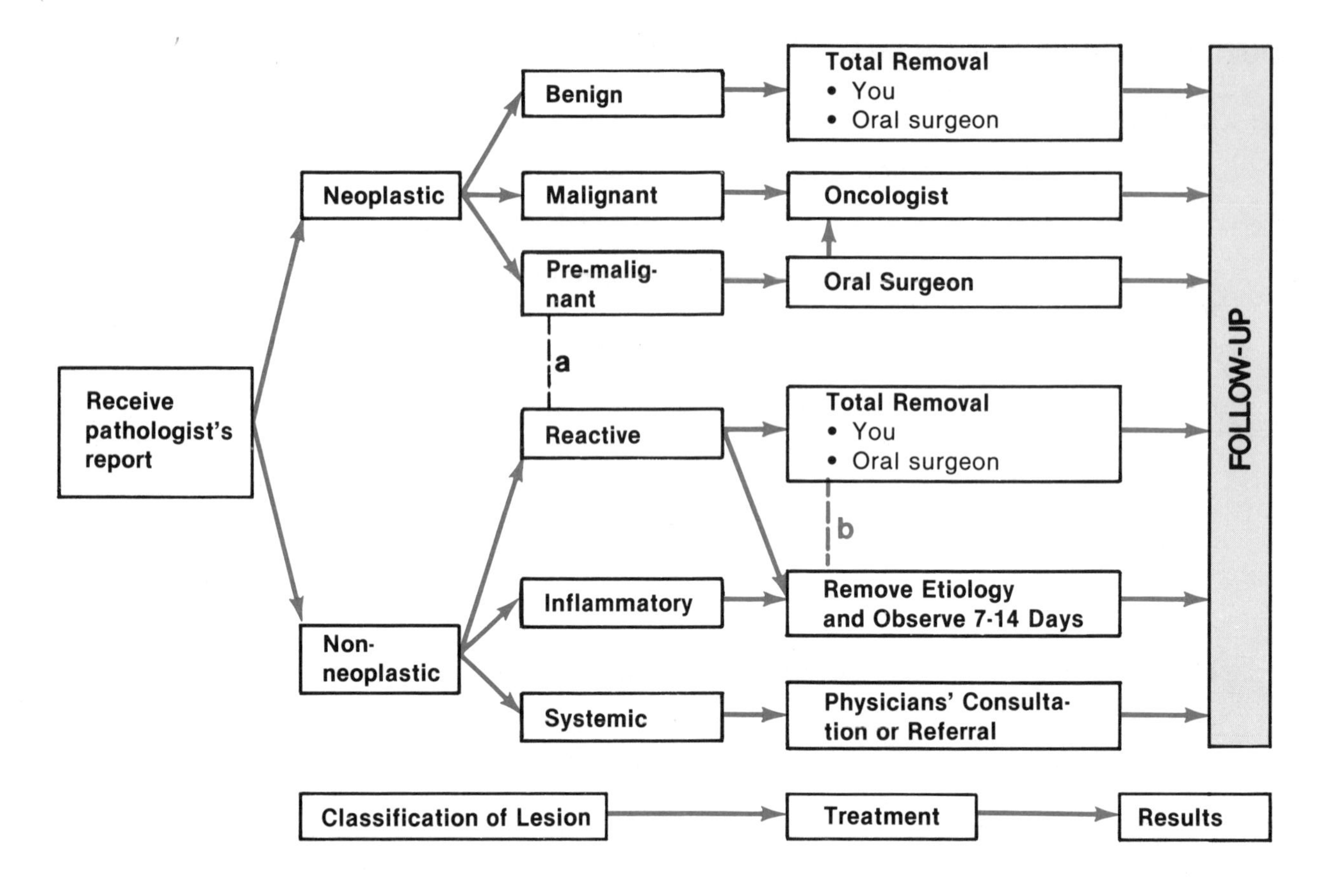

Figure IV-1. Flow Diagram for Management Options for Oral Lesions Based upon your Pathologist's Report. Black dashed line (a) represents the possibility of a concurrent occurrence of both a reactive and neoplastic process. Blue dashed line (b) implies that if lesion does not resolve following removal of probable etiology then total removal is indicated.

☐ **Malignant**

If the lesion is malignant, then you should IMMEDIATELY refer your patient to your local oncologist, or refer your patient to your oral surgeon. Your oral surgeon will likely consult with a tumor board. He may ask you to assist him with a description of the dental history and oral findings during a tumor board conference.

☐ **Pre-malignant**

Along with known neoplastic lesions, this category includes all dysplastic epithelial changes. If the lesion is diagnosed as pre-malignant, then you should refer your patient to your oral surgeon. Your oral surgeon will review the slides and pathology report and render the necessary service to the patient, usually total wide removal of any remaining lesion.

- **Non-neoplastic Lesions**

If the lesion is **non-neoplastic**, you must determine from the pathology report whether it is **reactive, inflammatory,** or **systemic** in nature. The terms commonly used in the pathology report for reactive lesions are summarized in the "terminology" section of this unit. Inflammatory lesions will usually be described in those words in the report. Lesions resulting from systemic conditions will usually be described as such. If in doubt, call your pathologist.

If the lesion is **reactive** in nature but has **epithelial changes,** complete removal is usually indicated. You may want to remove the lesion yourself or refer to an oral surgeon, based on your evaluation of the degree of difficulty.

If the lesion is **reactive** or **inflammatory**, you will want to remove the etiologic factor(s), if identified, and observe the lesion for a short period of time (not longer than 14 days).

If the lesion is the result of a **systemic condition** (such as diabetes, nutritional deficiencies, aging, medications for other medical problems, or hormonal imbalances), the tissue may reveal non-specific histopathologic data which must be interpreted along with clinical findings.

Keep in mind that if the biopsy report is not definitive or does not support your clinical opinion, you may elect to re-submit another tissue sample. The first tissue specimen you submitted may not be representative of the disease process. In such situations, a discussion with your pathologist will be helpful in planning future action.

All treatment avenues lead to the Follow-up Category where good periodic examinations are mandatory until the lesion has resolved. In the case of pre-malignant or malignant lesions, it may require continual follow-up for extended periods of time and occasionally for the rest of your patient's life.

STUDY EXERCISES—Unit IV

You have just received the following reports from your pathologist in the morning mail. Analyze each report as to the appropriate action required. Identify the key words in the report that clued your decisions.

Case #1

Microscopic Description: Sections contain a malignant epithelial neoplasm consisting of proliferating dyskeratotic epithelium which shows keratin pearl formation, abnormal mitosis, hyperchromatism, pleomorphism, and loss of polarity. The lesion extends to the lateral as well as the deep margins of the section.

Diagnosis: Incisional biopsy from right buccal mucosa: Well differentiated squamous cell carcinoma (Grade I WHO) (145.1).

Management of your case from here on: ______________________________

____

____

____

Key words of phrases: ______________________________

____

____

Case #2

Gross Description: The specimen consists of a 0.7 x 0.2 x 0.2 cm segment of mucosa.

Microscopic Description: The specimen consists of a segment of mucosa having hyperkeratinized and hyperparakeratinized epithelium. The epithelium is further marked by acanthosis with saw-tooth extension of rete pegs into the connective tissue. Mitotic figures are in evidence above those seen in normal epithelium. A small degree of dyskeratosis is noted in the epithelial cells. This takes the form of a small amount of keratinization at the lower cell levels. No other type of atypia is noted in the cells of the epithelium. The basal cell layer in many areas is difficult to visualize and micro-vesicles are apparent in the basement membrane space between the epithelium and the connective tissue. In some areas cleavage spaces are clearly noted between the epithelium and the connective tissue. Here no basal cell layer is noted in the epithelium and no basement membrane is noted between the two aspects of the tissue. The connective tissue is marked by a very prominent band of chronic inflammatory cells, primarily lymphocytes, which extend directly around the rete pegs of the epithelium. The lymphocytic infiltrate is a very dense one.

Pathologic Diagnosis: Lichen planus, buccal mucosa.

Comment: The specimen presents a classic case of lichen planus. All of the reported histologic findings are present here. Included among these is the presence of obvious cleavage between the epithelium and the connective tissue. Although no evidence of this was seen clinically, it would appear that such may well take place with time in this case. On a histologic basis then, a diagnosis of erosive lichen planus could be made on the basis of the obvious cleavage that is apparent at the histologic level. One additional note can be made. The dyskeratosis noted was a very minor amount of prekeratinization in some of the cells of the epithelium.

The second note is made to eliminate any possible thought of malignant process here. No evidence of malignancy is seen and no atypia other than that of this minor amount of dyskeratosis was noted.

Management of your case from here on: ______________________________

____

____

____

____

Key words or phrases: ______________________________

____

____

____

____

STUDY EXERCISES—Answers

Case #1

A. *Management*
This lesion is neoplastic and malignant. It should be referred to your local tumor board, oncologist or oral surgeon.

B. *Key words or phrases*
1. *Microscopic description words or phrases*

   a. *Malignant epithelial neoplasm*
   b. *Dyskeratotic epithelial cells*
   c. *Keratin pearls*
   d. *Abnormal mitosis*
   e. *Hyperchromatism*
   f. *Pleomorphism*
   g. *Loss of polarity*

2. *Diagnosis*

   a. *Well differentiated squamous cell carcinoma (Grade I)*

Case #2

A. *Management*
This lesion is non-neoplastic and inflammatory. You, as a general dentist, could treat it according to the treatment options described in your oral medicine or oral pathology training. If you do not have these management techniques in your "bag of tricks" refer your patient to an appropriate specialist.

B. *Key Words or Phrases*
1. *Microscopic Description Words or Phrases*

   a. *Hyperkeratinized*
   b. *Hyperparakeratinized epithelium*
   c. *Acanthosis*
   d. *Mitotic figures*
   e. *Small degree of dyskeratosis (keratinization in lower cell levels)*
   f. *Micro-vesicles in basement membrane—cleavage*
   g. *Prominent band of lymphocytes . . . rete pegs . . .*

2. *Diagnosis*

   a. *Lichen planus*

INFORMING YOUR PATIENT OF THE DIAGNOSIS

Informing the patient of a malignant diagnosis is a difficult task even for a trained oncologist. Unless the dentist knows the patient well, has good rapport and is confident that he/she knows the patient's psychological make-up, it may be better to depend on the family physician or the oral surgeon to inform the patient.

Information must be given positively, sincerely, and hopefully. The positive aspects of therapy and care should be emphasized. The terms "cancer" and "malignant" should be avoided, and the terms "growth" or "tumor" substituted.

When informing a patient of a malignant diagnosis, the patient will give the doctor clues concerning his/her need to know specific information. He/she will usually ask questions that he/she wants to know, thereby telling you the extent he/she wishes to be informed of his/her disease. If the doctor listens closely and responds accordingly, the task is made much easier.

Since many dentists are unfamiliar with this type of problem, it is always best to ask the family physician for help. He/she may prefer to inform the patient. The patient's family should also be informed of the diagnosis so they can support and assist the patient in obtaining treatment. Therefore, the following steps in informing the patient of a malignant diagnosis are advocated:

- Notify and discuss the psychological implications of the cancer diagnosis with the patient's family physician. He/she usually knows the patient's psychological make-up and may want to inform the patient.

- Make an appointment with the tumor board and/or an oncologist (surgeon or radiation therapist) who will carry out the treatment. The patient's family physician will usually help with these appointments.

- At the time the patient is informed of his cancer, preferably at the tumor board meeting, he/she must be told:
    a. That he/she has a growth or tumor.
    b. That this is how it will be treated.
        (1) Radiation and surgery
        (2) Surgery
        (3) Radiation
    c. Of his/her first appointment for treatment, either with the radiation therapist or the surgeon.

Very depressing news (psychologically damaging and frightening) has been given your patient. But hope and a way out of the problem have been provided by introducing the physicians who will outline the treatment and accomplish the therapy, and by scheduling the first appointment.

Usually it is best to tell the patient of his/her disease at the tumor board meeting or at least in conjunction with the oncologist where a complete treatment plan can be outlined.

REFERENCES

1. Batsakis, J. G.: **Tumors of the Head and Neck,** The Williams and Wilkens Company, Baltimore, 1974.
2. Bhaskar, S. N.: **Synopsis of Oral Pathology,** Fourth Edition, The C. V. Mosby Company, St. Louis, 1973.
3. Clark, H. B.: **Practical Oral Surgery,** Third Edition, Lea and Febiger, 1965.
4. Colby, R. A. Kerr, D. A., Robinson, H.B.G.: **Color Atlas of Oral Pathology,** Third Edition, J. B. Lippincott Company, Philadelphia, 1971.
5. Gorlin, R. J. and Goldman, H. M.: **Thoma's Oral Pathology,** Volume Two, The C. V. Mosby Company, 1970.
6. Kay, L. W. and Haskell, R.: **Color Atlas of Oro-Facial Diseases,** Year Book Medical Publishers, Inc., Chicago, 1971.
7. Kerr, D. A., Ash, Jr., M. M., Millard, H. D.: **Oral Diagnosis,** Fourth Edition, The C. V. Mosby Company, St. Louis, 1974.
8. Kruger, G. O.: **Textbook of Oral Surgery,** Third Edition, The C. V. Mosby Company, 1972.
9. Lumerman, H.: **Essentials of Oral Pathology,** J. B. Lippincott Company, Philadelphia, 1975.
10. Pindorg, J. J.: **Atlas of Diseases of the Oral Mucosa,** Second Edition, W. B. Saunders Company, Philadelphia, 1973.
11. Pindborg, J. J., Hjørting-Hansen, E.: **Atlas of Diseases of the Jaws,** W. B. Saunders Company, Philadelphia, 1974.
12. Shafer, Hines, and Levy: **Textbook of Oral Pathology,** Third Edition, W. B. Saunders Company, Philadelphia, 1974.
13. Sicher, H. and Bhaskar, S. N.: **Oral Histology and Embryology,** Seventh Edition, The C. V. Mosby Company, St. Louis, 1972.
14. Spouge, J. D.: **Oral Pathology,** The C. V. Mosby Company, St. Louis, 1973.
15. Waite, D. E.: **Textbook of Practical Oral Surgery,** Lea & Febiger, Philadelphia, 1972.
16. Wood, N. K. and Goat, P. W.: **Differential Diagnosis of Oral Lesions,** The C. V. Mosby Company, St. Louis, 1975.
17. Adams, R. S., Pullon, P. A., and Lee, F.: **Expanding the Role of the Dentist in the Detection of Oral and Laryngeal Cancer.** J. Am. Dent. Assoc. 89:607-610, 1974.
18. Bruun, J. P.: **Time Lapse by Diagnosis of Oral Cancer.** Oral Surgery, Oral Medicine, Oral Pathology, Vol. 42, Number 2, August 1976.

—Key—

Biopsy Evaluation
Summary of Factors

1. PATIENT'S GENERAL HEALTH

0—No history of medical problems or clinical conditions requiring modification in biopsy procedure.
1—History of medical problems which do not require a physician's consultation or modification of technique (i.e., drug allergies, some drug reactions, previous unrelated surgeries).
2—Medical history reveals conditions requiring a physician's consultation but **no modification** in surgical technique (i.e., rheumatic fever).
3—Medical history reveals conditions that require physician's consultation **and modification** of surgical technique (i.e., hemophilia, cardiovascular disease, etc.).

2. MALIGNANT POTENTIAL

0—No malignant potential.
1—The possibility of pre-malignancy is low in your differential diagnosis.
2—Pre-malignancy is a significant factor in your differential diagnosis.
3—High degree of malignant potential.

3. PHYSICAL PROPERTIES

A. **Definition of margins**
0—Well circumscribed with focal indistinct margins.
1—Indistinct margins.

B. **Surface Characteristics**
0—Surface contiguous with surrounding normal tissue.
1—Moderate irregular surface (compared to surrounding normal tissue).
2—Severe rough and/or irregular or ulcerated surface.

C. **Depth of Extension**
0—Superficial, involving epithelium and lamina propria.
1—Extending into connective tissue.
2—Extending into connective tissue and involving deeper structures, such as muscle, bone, fat, and salivary glands.

D. **Quality of Lesion**
0—Tissue normal quality (No B)
1—Less than 50% of the diameter of the lesion is of poor quality—$B/A \leq 50\%$
2—More than 50% of the diameter of the lesion is of poor quality—$B/A \geq 50\%$

E. **Pigmentation**
0—Non-pigmented.
1—Pigmentation of long standing or definite extrinsic etiology (amalgam tattoo).
2—No rating.
3—Pigmentation of short history or sudden change in color or size.

F. **Vascularity**
0—No abnormal vascular component.
1—Associated hyperemia.
2—Abnormal vascular component within lesion (angiofibroma).
3—Lesion entirely vascular in nature (hemangiomas, vascular hamartomas).

G. **Soft Tissue or Bone**
0—Soft tissue.
1—Soft tissue beginning to erode bone.
2—Soft tissue and bone involvement.
3—Entirely bony (central) lesion.

H. **Growth Rate**
0—No growth.
1—Slow growth (months to years).
2—Moderate growth (weeks to months).
3—Rapid growth (days to weeks)

I. **Overall Effect of Physical Properties**
0—All ratings in the "0" category.
1—All ratings in the "0" or "1" category.
2—All ratings in the "0" or "1" or "2" category (if more than two "2"s, this should be a "3").
3—Any "3"s plus more than two "2"s.

4. SIZE

0—Less than 0.5 cm (excisional biopsy technique).
1—0.5-1.0 cm (excisional biopsy technique).
2—1.0 cm + requiring only one incisional biopsy and lesions well localized.
3—1.0 cm + requiring multiple incisional biopsies (lesion not well localized and irregular in texture and outline).

5. DEGREE OF SURGICAL ACCESS

A. **Ability to See**
0—Direct unobstructed vision.
1—Requires minor manipulation of tissue or patient position.
2—Indirect vision with a mirror **or** tongue or cheek retraction.
3—Indirect vision with mirror required **as well** as retraction of tongue or cheek.

B. **Ability to Reach the Lesion**
0—Direct unobstructed instrument approach possible.
1—Requires minor manipulation of tissues or patient position in order to reach lesion with a direct approach.
2—Minor tongue or cheek retraction **or** slight modifications in surgical technique required to reach the lesion.
3—Major tissue or tongue retraction necessary **as well** as modifications in normal instrument utilization.

C. **Ability to Stabilize the Lesion**
0—Tissue not mobile, attached gingiva or hard palate.
1—Movable tissue with underlying bone-alveolar mucosa.
2—Soft tissue that can be easily immobilized by the operator—lips, buccal mucosa (cheek), anterior one-third of the tongue.
3—Very difficult to stabilize tissue, requires modification in basic technique. Soft palate, floor of mouth, ventral surface of tongue, anterior pillars.

D. **Underlying Anatomy**
0—No significant underlying structures (attached gingivae on mandible anterior to second molar and buccal of maxillary arch).
1—Underlying anatomic structures that would not preclude surgery in that area (buccal mucosa, lower lip, dorsal surface of tongue).
2—Significant anatomic structures and modification of surgical technique, i.e., around mental nerve, greater palatine foramen incisive canal, lesion in bone close to inferior alveolar bone.
3—Multiple significant adjacent anatomic structures located within the surgical bed which could cause permanent injury or a surgical emergency (i.e., incising the facial artery), or the lesion involves major anatomic structures (floor of the mouth contains nerves, blood vessels, salivary ducts, muscle attachments)

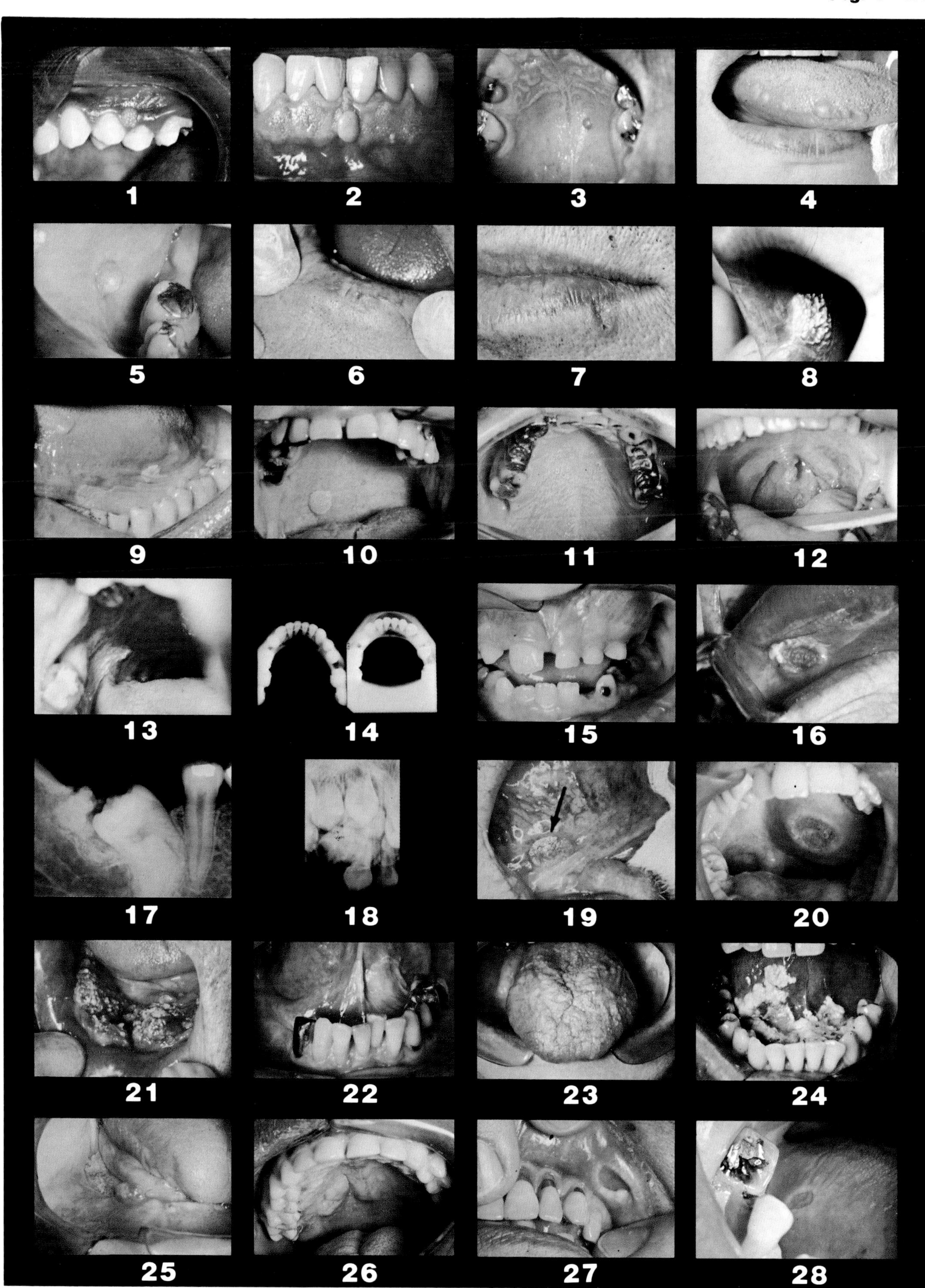
1
2
3
4
5
6
7
8
9
10
11
12
13
14
15
16
17
18
19
20
21
22
23
24
25
26
27
28

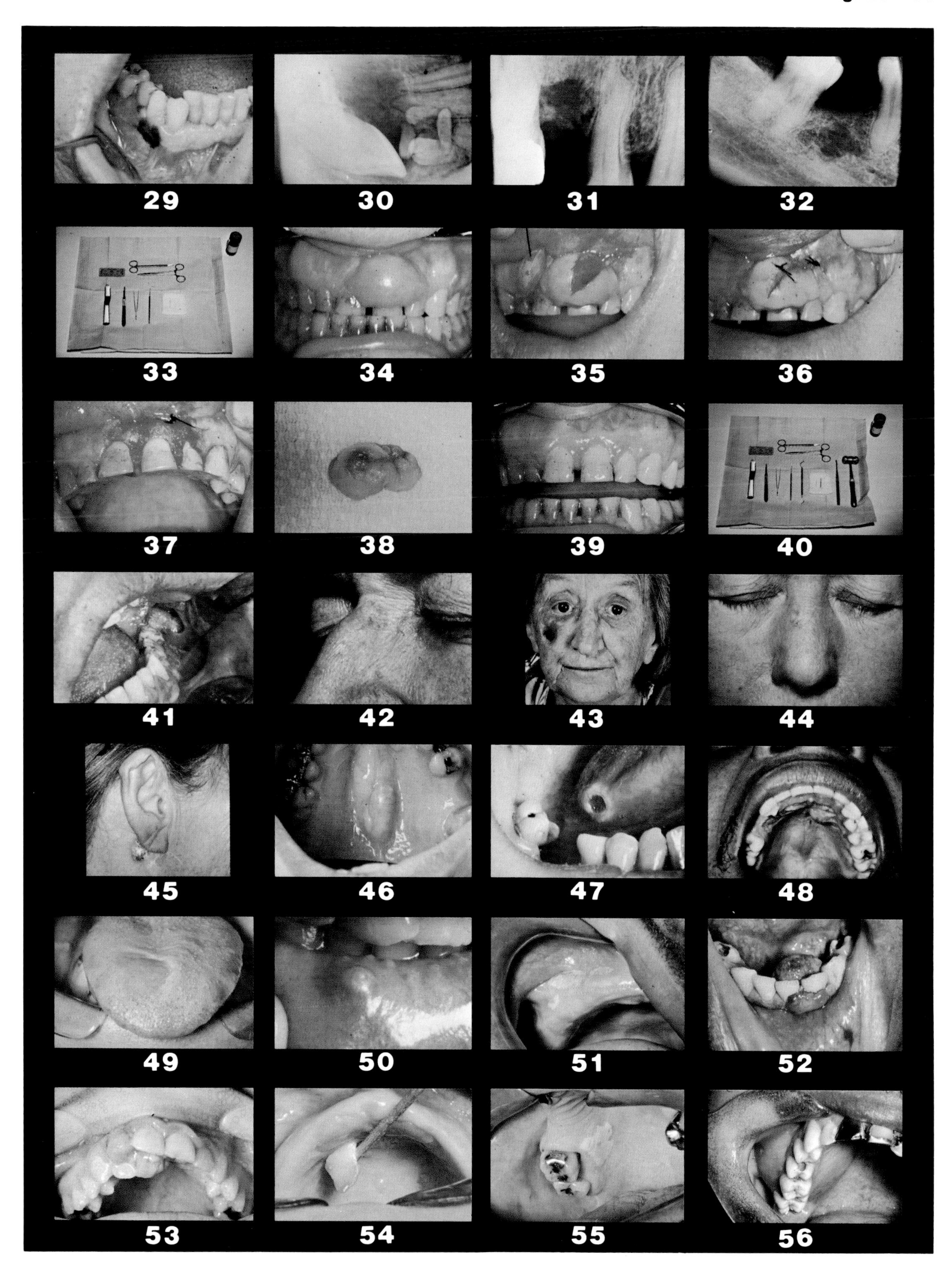
29
30
31
32
33
34
35
36
37
38
39
40
41
42
43
44
45
46
47
48
49
50
51
52
53
54
55
56

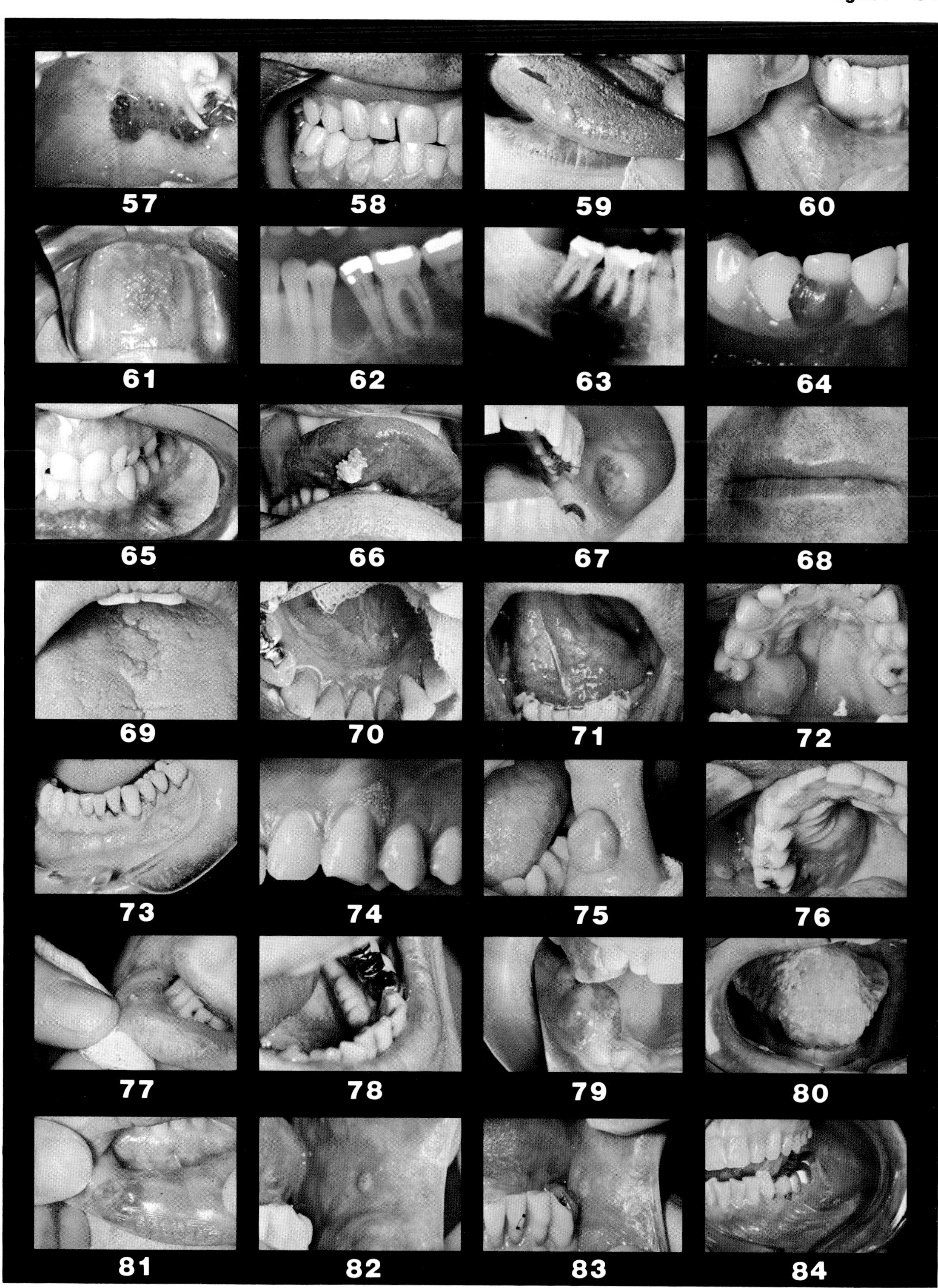
57
58
59
60
61
62
63
64
65
66
67
68
69
70
71
72
73
74
75
76
77
78
79
80
81
82
83
84

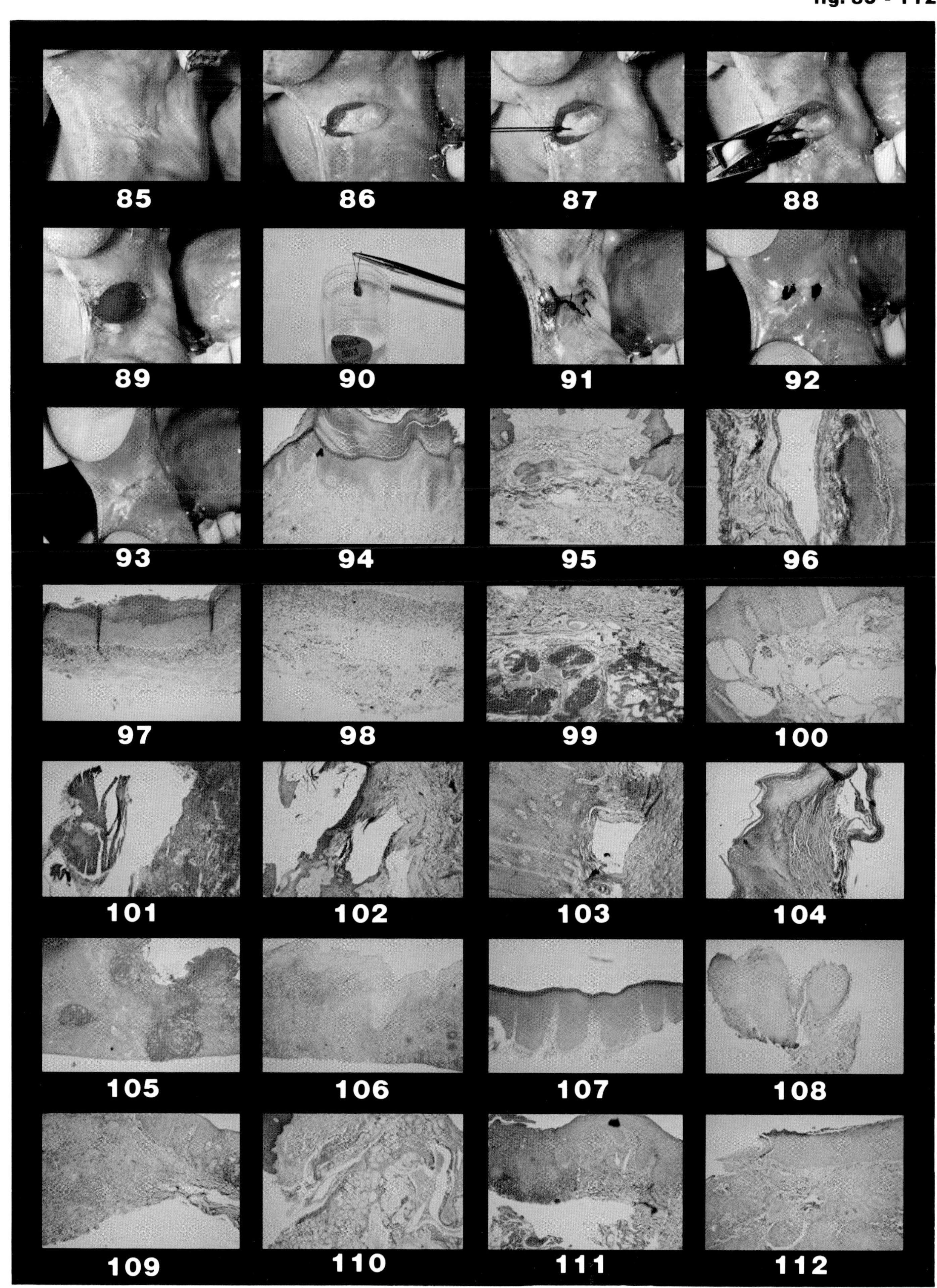
85
86
87
88
89
90
91
92
93
94
95
96
97
98
99
100
101
102
103
104
105
106
107
108
109
110
111
112

—Key—

Biopsy Evaluation
Summary of Factors

1. PATIENT'S GENERAL HEALTH

0—No history of medical problems or clinical conditions requiring modification in biopsy procedure.
1—History of medical problems which do not require a physician's consultation or modification of technique (i.e., drug allergies, some drug reactions, previous unrelated surgeries).
2—Medical history reveals conditions requiring a physician's consultation but **no modification** in surgical technique (i.e., rheumatic fever).
3—Medical history reveals conditions that require physician's consultation **and modification** of surgical technique (i.e., hemophilia, cardiovascular disease, etc.).

2. MALIGNANT POTENTIAL

0—No malignant potential.
1—The possibility of pre-malignancy is low in your differential diagnosis.
2—Pre-malignancy is a significant factor in your differential diagnosis.
3—High degree of malignant potential.

3. PHYSICAL PROPERTIES

A. **Definition of margins**
0—Well circumscribed with focal indistinct margins.
1—Indistinct margins.

B. **Surface Characteristics**
0—Surface contiguous with surrounding normal tissue.
1—Moderate irregular surface (compared to surrounding normal tissue).
2—Severe rough and/or irregular or ulcerated surface.

C. **Depth of Extension**
0—Superficial, involving epithelium and lamina propria.
1—Extending into connective tissue.
2—Extending into connective tissue and involving deeper structures, such as muscle, bone, fat, and salivary glands.

D. **Quality of Lesion**
0—Tissue normal quality (No B)
1—Less than 50% of the diameter of the lesion is of poor quality—B/A≤50%
2—More than 50% of the diameter of the lesion is of poor quality—B/A≥50%

E. **Pigmentation**
0—Non-pigmented.
1—Pigmentation of long standing or definite extrinsic etiology (amalgam tattoo).
2—No rating.
3—Pigmentation of short history or sudden change in color or size.

F. **Vascularity**
0—No abnormal vascular component.
1—Associated hyperemia.
2—Abnormal vascular component within lesion (angiofibroma).
3—Lesion entirely vascular in nature (hemangiomas, vascular hamartomas).

G. **Soft Tissue or Bone**
0—Soft tissue.
1—Soft tissue beginning to erode bone.
2—Soft tissue and bone involvement.
3—Entirely bony (central) lesion.

H. **Growth Rate**
0—No growth.
1—Slow growth (months to years).
2—Moderate growth (weeks to months).
3—Rapid growth (days to weeks)

I. **Overall Effect of Physical Properties**
0—All ratings in the "0" category.
1—All ratings in the "0" or "1" category.
2—All ratings in the "0" or "1" or "2" category (if more than two "2"s, this should be a "3").
3—Any "3"s plus more than two "2"s.

4. SIZE

0—Less than 0.5 cm (excisional biopsy technique).
1—0.5-1.0 cm (excisional biopsy technique).
2—1.0 cm + requiring only one incisional biopsy and lesions well localized.
3—1.0 cm + requiring multiple incisional biopsies (lesion not well localized and irregular in texture and outline).

5. DEGREE OF SURGICAL ACCESS

A. **Ability to See**
0—Direct unobstructed vision.
1—Requires minor manipulation of tissue or patient position.
2—Indirect vision with a mirror **or** tongue or cheek retraction.
3—Indirect vision with mirror required **as well** as retraction of tongue or cheek.

B. **Ability to Reach the Lesion**
0—Direct unobstructed instrument approach possible.
1—Requires minor manipulation of tissues or patient position in order to reach lesion with a direct approach.
2—Minor tongue or cheek retraction **or** slight modifications in surgical technique required to reach the lesion.
3—Major tissue or tongue retraction necessary **as well** as modifications in normal instrument utilization.

C. **Ability to Stabilize the Lesion**
0—Tissue not mobile, attached gingiva or hard palate.
1—Movable tissue with underlying bone-alveolar mucosa.
2—Soft tissue that can be easily immobilized by the operator—lips, buccal mucosa (cheek), anterior one-third of the tongue.
3—Very difficult to stabilize tissue, requires modification in basic technique. Soft palate, floor of mouth, ventral surface of tongue, anterior pillars.

D. **Underlying Anatomy**
0—No significant underlying structures (attached gingivae on mandible anterior to second molar and buccal of maxillary arch).
1—Underlying anatomic structures that would not preclude surgery in that area (buccal mucosa, lower lip, dorsal surface of tongue).
2—Significant anatomic structures and modification of surgical technique, i.e., around mental nerve, greater palatine foramen incisive canal, lesion in bone close to inferior alveolar bone.
3—Multiple significant adjacent anatomic structures located within the surgical bed which could cause permanent injury or a surgical emergency (i.e., incising the facial artery), or the lesion involves major anatomic structures (floor of the mouth contains nerves, blood vessels, salivary ducts, muscle attachments)

Evaluation and Treatment Record for Oral Lesions

Patient's Name ______________________

Address ______________________

____

Date lesion initially detected ______________

Your Name ______________

Address ______________

Phone Number ______________

Initial Action Required:

☐ 1. Observe for 7-14 days
☐ 2. Non-surgical treatment
☐ 3. Request laboratory tests
☐ 4. Malignant potential high—biopsy now
☐ 5. Make decision to biopsy

Histologic Examination Required: ☐ Yes ☐ No

Method

☐ Incisional ☐ Bone
☐ Excisional ☐ Aspiration
☐ Other: ______________

Pre-Surgical Evaluation:

	0	1	2	3	Comments
1. Patient's general health	☐	☐	☐	☐	
2. Malignant potential	☐	☐	☐	☐	
3. Physical properties					
A. Definition of margins	☐	☐	☐		
B. Surface characteristics	☐	☐	☐		
C. Depth of extension	☐	☐	☐		
D. Quality of tissue	☐	☐	☐		
E. Pigmentation	☐	☐	☐	☐	
F. Vascularity	☐	☐	☐	☐	
G. Soft tissue or bone	☐	☐	☐	☐	
H. Growth rate	☐	☐	☐	☐	
I. Overall effect of physical properties	☐	☐	☐	☐	
4. Size of lesion	☐	☐	☐	☐	
5. Degree of surgical access					
A. Ability to see	☐	☐	☐	☐	
B. Ability to reach	☐	☐	☐	☐	
C. Ability to stabilize	☐	☐	☐	☐	
D. Underlying anatomy	☐	☐	☐	☐	
6. OVERALL DIFFICULTY	☐	☐	☐	☐	

Who Did Surgery?

☐ I did
☐ Referred to ______________________

____

To Whom Was Specimen Submitted?

____

Date:

____

Pathologist's Report Received:

Date: ______________________

Comments:

☐ **Neoplastic**
- ☐ Benign
- ☐ Malignant
- ☐ Pre-malignant

☐ **Non-Neoplastic**
- ☐ Reactive
- ☐ Inflammatory
- ☐ Systemic

Course of Action

Referral to:

☐ Tumor board and oncologist:

____

☐ Oral surgeon:

____

☐ Physician:

____

My Treatment:

☐ Total removal
☐ Remove etiology
☐ Other: ______________________

Treatment Results: ______________________

____

____

Follow-Up Results: ______________________

____

____

____